そのまま使える
医療英会話

CD付

聖路加国際大学名誉教授
仁木久恵

筑波大学医学医療系准教授
森島祐子

筑波大学医学医療系准教授
F. Miyamasu

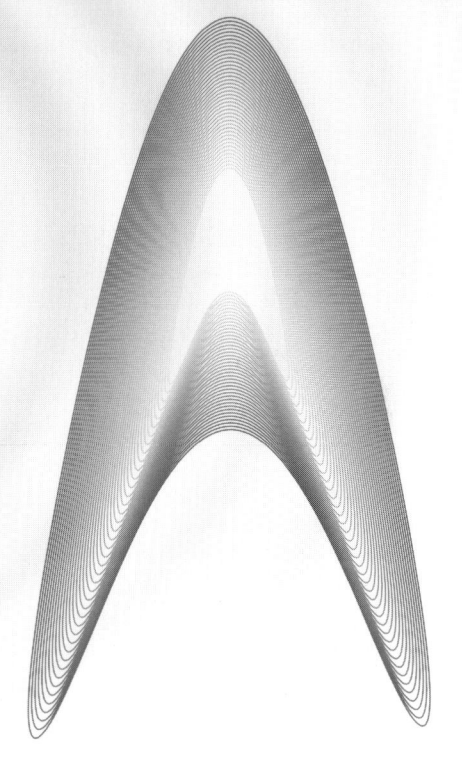

医学書院

著者紹介

仁木　久恵（にき　ひさえ）
　米国テキサス大学大学院にて M.A. 取得後，津田塾大学大学院博士課程修了．元 NHK ラジオ基礎英語講師．聖路加国際大学・明海大学教授を経て，現在，聖路加国際大学名誉教授．著書・訳書として『平静の心』（共訳：日野原重明），『臨床看護英語』（共著：Nancy Sharts-Hopko・横田まり子）など．

森島　祐子（もりしま　ゆうこ）
　米国生まれ．筑波大学医学専門学群在学中，カナダのマギル大学，マックマスター大学にて Clinical Clerkship を行う．医学博士．米国内科学会フェロー（FACP）．現在，筑波大学医学医療系准教授．専門分野は呼吸器病学．著書として『そのまま使える病院英語表現 5000』（共著：仁木久恵・Nancy Sharts-Hopko），『医療英会話キーワード辞典』（共著：仁木久恵・Flaminia Miyamasu）．

Flaminia Miyamasu（フラミニア　みやます）
　英国出身．リバプール大学卒業後，米国ジョージア大学大学院にて M.A. 取得（ロマンス諸語）．現在，筑波大学医学医療系准教授．専門分野は医学英語教育法．

そのまま使える医療英会話 ［CD 付］

発　行　2010 年 3 月 1 日　第 1 版第 1 刷©
　　　　2023 年 11 月 1 日　第 1 版第 5 刷
著　者　仁木久恵・森島祐子・Flaminia Miyamasu
発行者　株式会社　医学書院
　　　　代表取締役　金原　俊
　　　　〒113-8719　東京都文京区本郷 1-28-23
　　　　電話　03-3817-5600（社内案内）

印刷・製本　三美印刷

本書の複製権・翻訳権・上映権・譲渡権・貸与権・公衆送信権（送信可能化権を含む）は株式会社医学書院が保有します．

ISBN978-4-260-00878-5

本書を無断で複製する行為（複写，スキャン，デジタルデータ化など）は，「私的使用のための複製」など著作権法上の限られた例外を除き禁じられています．大学，病院，診療所，企業などにおいて，業務上使用する目的（診療，研究活動を含む）で上記の行為を行うことは，その使用範囲が内部的であっても，私的使用には該当せず，違法です．また私的使用に該当する場合であっても，代行業者等の第三者に依頼して上記の行為を行うことは違法となります．

[JCOPY]〈出版者著作権管理機構　委託出版物〉
本書の無断複製は著作権法上での例外を除き禁じられています．複製される場合は，そのつど事前に，出版者著作権管理機構（電話 03-5244-5088，FAX 03-5244-5089，info@jcopy.or.jp）の許諾を得てください．

本書の特色と活用法

①医療現場でそのまま使える
セクションAでは，医療スタッフが出会う様々なコミュニケーション場面を想定し，診療科別の会話に焦点を当てて編集しました．セクションBでは，診療科に特化した重要な表現が提示されています．情報収集のための質問や患者さんへの説明・指示表現を中心に取り上げましたので，CDの音声を聴きながら繰り返し練習して自分のものにして下さい．

②興味や必要に応じて，どの章からでも学習を始められる
各レッスンはそれぞれ独立した内容になっています．最初から取り組むのが理想的ですが，皆さんが関心をもつ診療科のレッスンから練習を始めてもかまいません．その場合，ご自分の診療科をマスターしてから他のレッスンへと進み，例文の一部を自分がよく使う単語に置き換えて応用して下さい．

③段階式に病院英会話の実践トレーニングを目指す
CDを聴いて状況にあった表現をインプットし，自分で声に出して言ってみる，さらにそれを応用するという流れを追っていくうちに，「話す力」が着実に身に付くように工夫してあります．

各レッスンの構成と使い方

Let's Listen!
患者さんとの間でかわされる自然な英語は，どのように聞こえるのでしょうか．CDの音声を聴いて，英語独特のリズム，会話の流れや間の取り方，そして英語的な発想に慣れて下さい．最初はテキストを見てもけっこうですが，内容を理解してからはテキストを閉じて聴くとよいでしょう．

CDのマーク，数字はトラックナンバーです．

色字は医療スタッフが使う表現を示しています．

会話文の日本語訳です．必要に応じて参照して下さい．

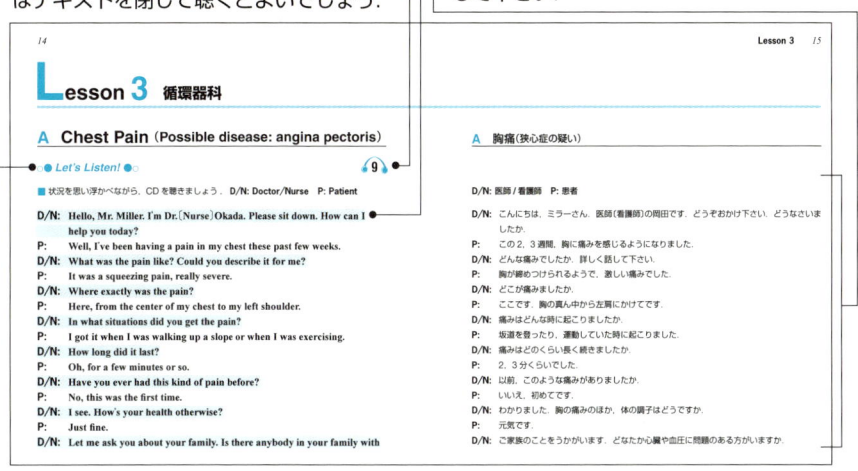

Words & Phrases

次のステップのための準備練習．一つひとつの語句を正確に発音できるように，CDの音声を聴いて必ず声に出して言ってみましょう．

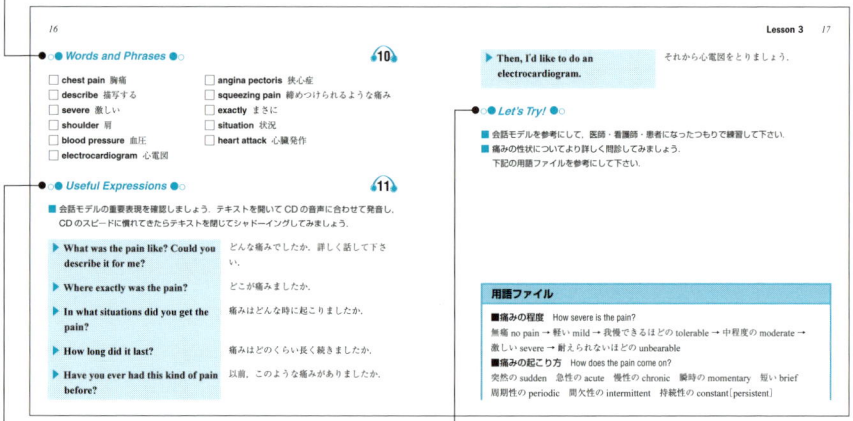

Useful Expressions

話すための実践トレーニング．

シャドーイングとは，CDの音声を聴きながら，「影」のようにその後を追いかけて発音してゆく語学訓練法の一つです．会話のスピードに慣れていくうちに，「聴く力」と「話す力」の両方をアップさせます．

① 初めは，テキストを見ながらCDのスピードに合わせて声に出して言ってみます．自分の声でCDの音声が聴こえないこともあるので，ヘッドフォンをつけたり，または音量をあげるとよいでしょう．

② シャドーイングをします．テキストを見ないで，CDの音声の後について医療スタッフのセリフの部分を声に出して言ってみましょう．途中で聴きそこなった語句があっても，そこで立ち止まらずに，どんどん流れてくるCDの音声のほうに集中して下さい．初めは口がついていかないかもしれませんが，慣れていくうちに英語のリズムやイントネーションを体得することができるでしょう．

Let's Try!

Let's Listen! の会話モデルに沿って，医療スタッフ役と患者役に分かれてロールプレイして下さい．患者役の人はテキストを見てもよいでしょう．個人で学習する場合，ひとり二役を演じるのは難しいかもしれませんが，患者役のほうは黙読して，医療スタッフ役のセリフを声に出して言ってみましょう．

次に，会話モデルにとらわれることなく，臨床の場で出会うであろう様々な状況を想定したシナリオを作って，自由に話し合ってみましょう．用語ファイルをヒントに会話が発展するよう，積極的に取り組んで下さい．「話す力」を身につけるには，声に出して言ってみること，そして楽しみながら継続していくことが大切です．

記号

〔 〕は，その直前の語(句)と入れ替え可能であることを示す．

[ ]は，その直前の語(句)と同義であることを示す．

( )は，省略可能であることを示す．

なお，本書は『そのまま使える病院英語表現5000』(医学書院)の実践編として編まれました．医療の現場で通用する語彙や表現，そして情報量をさらにアップするために，合わせてご利用いただければ幸いです．

外国人患者との効果的なコミュニケーション 10 か条

1. 初診時には自己紹介し,患者の名前を言って確かめる.
2. コンピュータ画面やカルテから目を離して,患者と目を合わせながら話す.
3. 自分のほうから声をかけて笑顔で接する.患者の気持ちを和らげるように努力する.
4. ゆっくり,そしてはっきり話す.患者の母語が英語であるとはかぎらない.
5. 平易な英語で話し,専門用語はなるべく使わない.
6. 必要に応じてジェスチャーを使う.イラストや資料を用いて説明する.
7. 患者が話す内容を正確に把握するために,重要な情報は再確認する.
8. 診察や検査を行う前にはきちんと説明する.
9. 自分が話した内容を患者に繰り返し言ってもらい,情報が正確に伝わったかを確認する.
10. 患者が退室するときには目を合わせて挨拶をする.

最後に,患者との信頼関係を築くために医療従事者も'**patient**'であること.

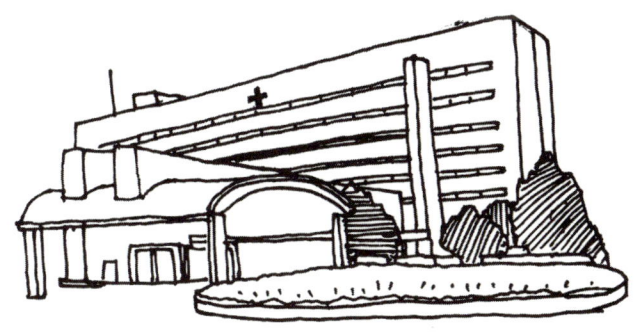

目次

Lesson 1　患者さんのプロフィールを訊く　2
　　A. 診療科の受付で　2
　　B. 個人に関する一般情報　6

Lesson 2　診察室に患者さんを迎える　8
　　A. 診察室でのあいさつ　8
　　B. 病歴をとるためのヒント　12

Lesson 3　循環器科　14
　　A. 胸痛（狭心症の疑い）　14
　　B. バイタルサインと心電図　18

Lesson 4　呼吸器科　20
　　A. 咳・熱・頭痛（急性気管支炎の疑い）　20
　　B. 胸背部の診察　24

Lesson 5　消化器科　26
　　A. 腹痛（急性胃炎の疑い）　26
　　B. 腹部の診察/内視鏡検査　31

Lesson 6　代謝・内分泌科　34
　　A. 健診異常（糖尿病の疑い）　34
　　B. 尿検査と血液検査　38

Lesson 7　救急　40
　　A. 頭部外傷　40
　　B. X線検査とCT・MRI検査　44

Lesson 8　泌尿器科　48
　　A. 背部痛・血尿（腎結石の疑い）　48
　　B. 超音波検査（エコー）　52

Lesson 9	乳腺外科　54	
	A. 乳房のしこり（乳癌の疑い）　54	
	B. 手術の説明　59	
Lesson 10	脳神経科　60	
	A. めまい（脳出血の疑い）　60	
	B. 入院　65	
Lesson 11	心療内科・精神科　68	
	A. 疲労・体重減少・睡眠障害（適応障害の疑い）　68	
	B. 薬剤投与　72	
Lesson 12	皮膚科　74	
	A. 湿疹（アトピー性皮膚炎の疑い）　74	
	B. アレルギー歴　79	
Lesson 13	産婦人科　80	
	A. 妊娠　80	
	B. 産科診察　85	
Lesson 14	小児科　88	
	A. 喘息発作　88	
	B. 予防接種・健診　92	
Lesson 15	会計窓口　94	
	A. 診療費の支払い　94	
	B. 保険・支払い　98	
Lesson 16	病院のなかの基礎用語　100	
	1. 診療部門　100	
	2. 病院関係者　102	
	3. 病名　104	

索引　109

本文イラスト：大日方 謙介

●用語ファイル
- ■言葉の問題について　5
- ■患者の話を確認するために　11
- ■痛みの程度，痛みの起こり方，痛みの頻度　17
- ■咳の種類，咳の程度，痰の種類，痰の色　23
- ■便の形・硬さ，便の色，便の臭い　30
- ■貧血の一般的な徴候　37
- ■手足の怪我　43
- ■膀胱炎の一般的な症状　51
- ■月経についての情報　58
- ■メニエール病の一般的な症状　64
- ■パニック発作の一般的な症状　71
- ■花粉症の一般的な症状　78
- ■つわりの一般的な症状　84
- ■水痘・風疹の一般的な症状　91
- ■処方箋について　97

●スピーキング攻略のヒント
- （1）英語のリズム　25
- （2）イントネーション（声の抑揚）　47
- （3）音の連結　53
- （4）音の脱落　67
- （5）品詞による発音の違い　87

●コラム
- 腹痛または胃痛，どっちなの？　33
- 頻度の表現　73
- 医学専門用語と一般語　99

そのまま使える医療英会話

Lesson 1　患者さんのプロフィールを訊く

A　At Reception

○● *Let's Listen!* ●○

■ 状況を思い浮かべながら，CD を聴きましょう． **N/C: Nurse/Clerk　P: Patient**

N/C:	Good morning. Is this your first visit?
P:	Yes, it is.
N/C:	Then, please fill out this form. Write in block letters, please.
P:	All right.
	………
P:	I'm finished. Here it is.
N/C:	Thank you. Well, how do you pronounce your last name?
P:	MacGuire.
N/C:	I beg your pardon?
P:	MacGuire.
N/C:	Mac... I'm sorry, I still didn't catch your name. Could you pronounce it again more slowly?
P:	Sure. *Mac-Guire* … *Ma-gwire*.
N/C:	Thank you, Mr. MacGuire. Who sent you to our office?
P:	Dr. Hayashi, my family doctor.
N/C:	Do you have a referral letter from him?
P:	Yes, here you are.
N/C:	The doctor will see you soon. Could you wait here until we call your name?
P:	Sure.
N/C:	Please let us know if you feel sick.
P:	Thank you. I'm OK right now.
	………
N/C:	Mr. MacGuire, please come into Room 2. This way, please.

A 診療科の受付で

N/C: 看護師 / クラーク　**P:** 患者

N/C: おはようございます．初診ですか．
P: はい，そうです．
N/C: それでは，この用紙にご記入下さい．活字体で書いて下さい．
P: わかりました．
　　　………
P: 書き終わりました．はい，どうぞ．
N/C: ありがとう．ところで，姓のほうのお名前はどう発音するのですか．
P: マクガイヤです．
N/C: もう一度言って下さい．
P: マクガイヤです．
N/C: マック…ごめんなさい．お名前が聞き取れなかったので，もう一度ゆっくり発音していただけませんか．
P: ええ，いいですよ．マクガイヤ，マ・ガイヤ．
N/C: はい，マクガイヤさんですね．どなたのご紹介ですか．
P: かかりつけ医の林先生です．
N/C: 紹介状をお持ちですか．
P: はい，これです．
N/C: もうすぐドクターが診察します．お名前をお呼びするまでここでお待ち下さい．

P: はい．
N/C: ご気分が悪かったらおっしゃって下さい．
P: ありがとう．今は大丈夫です．
　　　………
N/C: マクガイヤさん，2番の診察室にお入り下さい．こちらへどうぞ．

○● Words and Phrases ●○

- [ ] first visit　初診
- [ ] form　用紙
- [ ] thank you　ありがとう
- [ ] pardon　もう一度言って
- [ ] Could you...?　していただけますか
- [ ] family doctor　かかりつけ医
- [ ] wait　待つ
- [ ] fill out　記入する
- [ ] block letters　活字体
- [ ] pronounce　発音する
- [ ] I'm sorry　ごめんなさい
- [ ] again　もう一度
- [ ] referral letter　紹介状
- [ ] feel sick　気分が悪い

○● Useful Expressions ●○

■ 会話モデルの重要表現を確認しましょう．テキストを開いてCDの音声に合わせて発音し，CDのスピードに慣れてきたらテキストを閉じてシャドーイングしてみましょう．

▶ Good morning.	おはようございます．
▶ Is this your first visit?	初診ですか．
▶ Then, please fill out this form.	それでは，この用紙にご記入下さい．
▶ Write in block letters, please.	活字体で書いて下さい．
▶ How do you pronounce your last name?	姓のほうのお名前はどう発音するのですか．
▶ I beg your pardon?	もう一度言って下さい．
▶ I'm sorry, I still didn't catch your name.	ごめんなさい．お名前が聞き取れませんでした．
▶ Could you pronounce it again more slowly?	もう一度ゆっくり発音していただけませんか．
▶ Who sent you to our office?	どなたのご紹介ですか．
▶ Do you have a referral letter from him?	紹介状をお持ちですか．
▶ The doctor will see you soon.	もうすぐドクターが診察します．

▶ Could you wait here until we call your name?	お名前をお呼びするまでここでお待ち下さい．
▶ Please let us know if you feel sick.	ご気分が悪かったらおっしゃって下さい．
▶ Mr. MacGuire, please come into Room 2. This way, please.	マクガイヤさん，2番の診察室にお入り下さい．こちらへどうぞ．

○● *Let's Try!* ●○

■ 会話モデルを参考にして，看護師・クラーク・患者になったつもりで練習して下さい．
■ 患者の日本語能力を尋ねる質問を会話の中に入れて練習してみましょう．
　下記の用語ファイルを参考にして下さい．

用語ファイル

■言葉の問題について

日本語が話せるか	Do you speak Japanese?*
日本語の読み書きができるか	Do you read and write Japanese?*
誰か日本語を話す人がいるか	Is there anyone who can speak Japanese?
—それは誰か	— Who is he〔she〕?
通訳を必要とするか	Do you need an intérpreter?**
母語は何か	What's your native language?

　　*日本語能力を尋ねる場合，Can you…? よりも Do you…? のほうが丁寧な言い方になる．
　　**ストレスマーク(´)のついた部分は強く発音する．

B Patient Profile　　個人に関する一般情報

■ 患者さんから正確なデータを得るための具体的な表現を集めました．テキストを開いてCDの音声に合わせて発音し，CDのスピードに慣れてきたらテキストを閉じてシャドーイングをしてみましょう．

🎧 **4**

▶ Can you tell me a little about yourself?　　いくつか質問をいたします．

▶ I'd like to ask you some questions.　　いくつか質問をいたします．

Name・Age　　名前・年齢

▶ What's your name, please?　　お名前をお聞かせ下さい．
   ● 上昇調でいう．

▶ May I have your name?　　お名前をお聞かせ下さい．
   ● より丁寧な表現．

▶ How do you spell your name?　　お名前はどうつづるのですか．
   ● 姓は family (last) name,
     個人名は first name.

▶ How old are you?　　年はおいくつですか．

▶ What's your date of birth?　　生年月日はいつですか．

▶ When were you born?　　生年月日はいつですか．

Birthplace・Nationality　　出生地・国籍

▶ Where are you from?　　ご出身はどちらですか．

▶ Where were you born?　　どこで生まれましたか．

▶ What's your place of birth?　　どこで生まれましたか．

▶ What's your nationality?　　国籍はどちらですか．

▶ When did you come to Japan? いつ日本へ来ましたか.

▶ How long have you stayed in Japan? 日本に住んでどのくらいになりますか.

▶ How long are you going to stay here? これからどのくらい滞在しますか.

Address・Phone number・Email address 　住所・電話番号・E メールアドレス

▶ Where do you live? どこにお住まいですか.

▶ What's your (home) address? 住所はどちらですか.

▶ What's your permanent address 〔business address〕? 本籍地〔勤務先の住所〕はどちらですか.

▶ What's your phone number〔business phone number〕? 自宅〔勤務先〕のお電話は何番ですか.

▶ What's your email address? E メールアドレスは何ですか.

▶ What's your emergency contact number? 緊急連絡先は何番ですか.

▶ Who is the person to be contacted in an emergency? 緊急連絡先はどなたですか.
— Can you tell me his〔her〕name and your relationship to him〔her〕? ―その方の名前，ご関係を教えて下さい.

Lesson 2　診察室に患者さんを迎える

A　Greetings

○● *Let's Listen!* ●○

■ 状況を思い浮かべながら，CD を聴きましょう．　D/N: Doctor/Nurse　P: Patient

（初診の場合）

D/N: Hello, I'm Dr.〔Nurse〕Mori. Are you Mrs. Bates?
P: That's right.
D/N: I'm sorry to have kept you waiting. Please sit down. How can I help you today?
P: I've been feeling dizzy.
D/N: I've just read the referral letter from Dr. Fujii. He says you've been having trouble with your heart.
P: Yes, that's right.
D/N: Tell me about it.
P: Sure. I've been short of breath, and...

（再診の場合）

D/N: Good morning, Ms. Baston.
P: Good morning, Doctor〔Nurse〕.
D/N: Nice to see you again. Sit down, please. How have you been since I last saw you?
P: Much better.
D/N: Did the last medication work well?
P: Yes, but I've lost my appetite, and I've also been troubled with constipation.
D/N: I'm sorry to hear that. Anything else?

A　診察室でのあいさつ

D/N: 医師／看護師　P: 患者

D/N:　こんにちは．私は医師〔看護師〕の森です．ベイツさんですね．
P:　　はい，そうです．
D/N:　お待たせしました．どうぞお座り下さい．どうなさいましたか．

P:　　めまいが続いているのです．
D/N:　藤井先生からの紹介状を読ませていただきました．先生によると心臓の具合が悪いのですね．
P:　　はい，そうです．
D/N:　そのことについてお話し下さい．
P:　　はい．息切れがして…

D/N:　バストンさん，おはようございます．
P:　　おはようございます．
D/N:　またお会いできてうれしいです．どうぞお座り下さい．この前診察してから具合はいかがですか．
P:　　ずっとよくなっています．
D/N:　この前の薬は効きましたか．
P:　　ええ，でも食欲がなくて，それに便秘でも困っています．

D/N:　それはいけませんね．そのほか何かありますか．

○● Words and Phrases ●○

- [ ] nurse 看護師
- [ ] sit down 座る
- [ ] have trouble with... 具合が悪い
- [ ] be short of breath 息切れする
- [ ] work well 効く
- [ ] constipation 便秘
- [ ] hello こんにちは
- [ ] feel dizzy めまいがする
- [ ] heart 心臓
- [ ] medication 薬
- [ ] appetite 食欲

○● Useful Expressions ●○

■ 会話モデルの重要表現を確認しましょう．テキストを開いて CD の音声に合わせて発音し，CD のスピードに慣れてきたらテキストを閉じてシャドーイングしてみましょう．

▶ Hello, I'm Dr. Mori.	こんにちは．私は医師の森です．
▶ Are you Mrs. Bates?	ベイツさんですね．
▶ I'm sorry to have kept you waiting. Please sit down.	お待たせしました．どうぞお座り下さい．
▶ How can I help you today?	どうなさいましたか．
▶ I've just read the referral letter from Dr. Fujii.	藤井先生からの紹介状を読ませていただきました．
▶ He says you've been having trouble with your heart.	先生によると心臓の具合が悪いのですね．
▶ Tell me about it.	そのことについてお話し下さい．
▶ Nice to see you again.	またお会いできてうれしいです．
▶ How have you been since I last saw you?	この前診察してから具合はいかがですか．
▶ Did the last medication work well?	この前の薬は効きましたか．
▶ I'm sorry to hear that.	それはいけませんね．
▶ Anything else?	そのほか何かありますか．

○● *Let's Try!* ●○

■ 会話モデルを参考にして，医師・看護師・患者になったつもりで練習して下さい．
■ 下記の用語ファイルを参考にして，患者の話を確認しながら会話をしてみましょう．

用語ファイル

■患者の話を確認するために

もう一度言ってほしい	（I beg your）pardon?　↗（上昇調でいう）
もっとゆっくり話してほしい	Could you speak more slowly?
もっとゆっくり発音してほしい	Could you pronounce it more slowly?
話をテープにとりたい	Is it all right if I use this tape recorder?
紙に書いてほしい	Could you write it on this paper?

B Clinical Hints (Wh Questions)　病歴をとるためのヒント

■ 患者さんから正確なデータを得るための具体的な表現を集めました．テキストを開いてCDの音声に合わせて発音し，CDのスピードに慣れてきたらテキストを閉じてシャドーイングをしてみましょう．

🎧 8

General Questions　一般的な質問

▶ (Do you have) any problems with your eyes (breathing/stomach/skin)?　目〔呼吸／胃／皮膚〕に何か問題がありますか．

Symptoms　症状について

1) 症状の特徴

▶ What is the problem like?　どんな症状ですか．

▶ What does it feel like?　どんな具合ですか．

▶ What kind of problem is it?　どんな種類の症状ですか．

▶ How severe is it?　程度はどれくらいですか．

2) 症状の部位

▶ Where is it?　場所はどこですか．

▶ Does it spread to other parts of the body?　放散しますか．

3) 経過

①発症時刻，時期

▶ When did it start?　いつ発症しましたか．

▶ When did you first notice it?　最初に気づいたのはいつですか．

▶ When does it usually come on?　たいていどんな時に起こりますか．

▶ At a specific time at night (in the morning)?　夜〔朝〕などの特に決まった時間帯ですか．

②症状の起こり方

▶ How does it come on? — どんな起こり方ですか．

▶ Suddenly or gradually? — 突然ですか，徐々にですか．

▶ Does it come and go, or does it stay? — 症状は一過性ですか，持続性ですか．

③持続時間，期間

▶ How long have you had it? — どのくらい続いていますか．

▶ How long does it last each time? — 毎回どのくらい続きますか．

④頻度

▶ How often does it occur? — 起こる頻度はどのくらいですか．

▶ How often do you have it? — 起こる頻度はどのくらいですか．

⑤症状の経過

▶ Is it getting better, getting worse, or is there no change? — 軽快傾向ですか，悪化傾向ですか，変化なしですか．

⑥同様の症状の経験

▶ Have you had this kind of symptom before? — このような症状を経験したことがありますか．

▶ When〔Where/By whom/How〕was it treated? — いつ〔どこで／誰から／どんな〕治療を受けましたか．

4) 症状の誘発因子，増悪因子，緩和因子

▶ What brings〔brought〕it on? — 何が原因で起こりますか〔起こりましたか〕．

▶ What do you think is〔was〕causing it? — 思い当たる誘因は何ですか．

▶ Is there any cause you can identify? — 思い当たる誘因がありますか．

▶ What makes it worse? — 悪化させるものは何ですか．

▶ What makes it better〔go away〕? — 緩和させる〔消す〕ものは何ですか．

5) 随伴症状

▶ Do you have any other signs or symptoms? — ほかに徴候や症状がありますか．

Lesson 3 循環器科

A Chest Pain (Possible disease: angina pectoris)

○● *Let's Listen!* ●○   9

■ 状況を思い浮かべながら，CD を聴きましょう．　D/N: Doctor/Nurse　P: Patient

D/N: Hello, Mr. Miller. I'm Dr.〔Nurse〕Okada. Please sit down. How can I help you today?

P: Well, I've been having a pain in my chest these past few weeks.

D/N: What was the pain like? Could you describe it for me?

P: It was a squeezing pain, really severe.

D/N: Where exactly was the pain?

P: Here, from the center of my chest to my left shoulder.

D/N: In what situations did you get the pain?

P: I got it when I was walking up a slope or when I was exercising.

D/N: How long did it last?

P: Oh, for a few minutes or so.

D/N: Have you ever had this kind of pain before?

P: No, this was the first time.

D/N: I see. How's your health otherwise?

P: Just fine.

D/N: Let me ask you about your family. Is there anybody in your family with heart or blood pressure trouble?

P: My father died when he was 52 of a heart attack. That was 10 years ago.

D/N: Anybody else?

P: No, but I've been wondering whether there's something wrong with my heart.
　　………

D: Well, let me listen to your heart. Then, I'd like to do an electrocardiogram.

A　胸痛（狭心症の疑い）

D/N: 医師／看護師　**P:** 患者

D/N: こんにちは，ミラーさん．医師〔看護師〕の岡田です．どうぞおかけ下さい．どうなさいましたか．
P: この2，3週間，胸に痛みを感じるようになりました．
D/N: どんな痛みでしたか．詳しく話して下さい．
P: 胸が締めつけられるようで，激しい痛みでした．
D/N: どこが痛みましたか．
P: ここです．胸の真ん中から左肩にかけてです．
D/N: 痛みはどんな時に起こりましたか．
P: 坂道を登ったり，運動していた時に起こりました．
D/N: 痛みはどのくらい長く続きましたか．
P: 2，3分くらいでした．
D/N: 以前，このような痛みがありましたか．
P: いいえ，初めてです．
D/N: わかりました．胸の痛みのほか，体の調子はどうですか．
P: 元気です．
D/N: ご家族のことをうかがいます．どなたか心臓や血圧に問題のある方がいますか．

P: 父が52歳のときに心臓発作で亡くなっています．10年前です．
D/N: ほかには？
P: いませんが，私は心臓が悪いのではないかと思っているのです．

　　　　………

D: それでは，心臓の聴診をします．それから心電図をとりましょう．

○● Words and Phrases ●○

- [ ] **chest pain** 胸痛
- [ ] **describe** 描写する
- [ ] **severe** 激しい
- [ ] **shoulder** 肩
- [ ] **blood pressure** 血圧
- [ ] **electrocardiogram** 心電図
- [ ] **angina pectoris** 狭心症
- [ ] **squeezing pain** 締めつけられるような痛み
- [ ] **exactly** まさに
- [ ] **situation** 状況
- [ ] **heart attack** 心臓発作

○● Useful Expressions ●○

■ 会話モデルの重要表現を確認しましょう．テキストを開いてCDの音声に合わせて発音し，CDのスピードに慣れてきたらテキストを閉じてシャドーイングしてみましょう．

▶ What was the pain like? Could you describe it for me?	どんな痛みでしたか．詳しく話して下さい．
▶ Where exactly was the pain?	どこが痛みましたか．
▶ In what situations did you get the pain?	痛みはどんな時に起こりましたか．
▶ How long did it last?	痛みはどのくらい長く続きましたか．
▶ Have you ever had this kind of pain before?	以前，このような痛みがありましたか．
▶ How's your health otherwise?	胸の痛みのほか，体の調子はどうですか．
▶ Let me ask you about your family.	ご家族のことをうかがいます．
▶ Is there anybody in your family with heart or blood pressure trouble?	どなたか心臓や血圧に問題のある方がいますか．
▶ Anybody else?	ほかには？
▶ Well, let me listen to your heart.	それでは，心臓の聴診をします．

▶ **Then, I'd like to do an electrocardiogram.**   それから心電図をとりましょう．

○● *Let's Try!* ●○

■ 会話モデルを参考にして，医師・看護師・患者になったつもりで練習して下さい．
■ 痛みの性状についてより詳しく問診してみましょう．
　下記の用語ファイルを参考にして下さい．

用語ファイル

■**痛みの程度**　How severe is the pain?
無痛 no pain → 軽い mild → 我慢できるほどの tolerable → 中程度の moderate → 激しい severe → 耐えられないほどの unbearable

■**痛みの起こり方**　How does the pain come on?
突然の sudden　急性の acute　慢性の chronic　瞬時の momentary　短い brief
周期性の periodic　間欠性の intermittent　持続性の constant [persistent]

■**痛みの頻度**　How often do you have the pain?
いつも always → たいてい usually → しばしば often → 頻繁に frequently →
繰り返し over and over → 時々 sometimes → まれに rarely

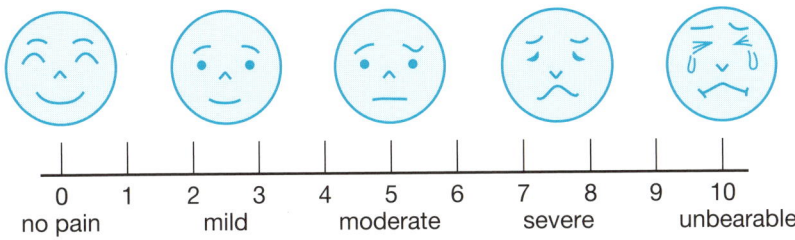

Please look at this scale of zero to ten. What's your pain level now?
0 から 10 の痛みのスケールをご覧下さい．あなたの今の痛みのレベルは何ですか．

B Vital Signs and ECG バイタルサインと心電図

■ 患者さんから正確なデータを得るための具体的な表現を集めました．テキストを開いてCDの音声に合わせて発音し，CDのスピードに慣れてきたらテキストを閉じてシャドーイングをしてみましょう．

🎧 12

Vital Signs / バイタルサイン

▶ I'm going to take your temperature.　熱［体温］を測りましょう．
— Please keep this thermometer under your arm for one minute.　―この体温計をわきの下に1分間はさんで下さい．
— Your temperature is thirty-seven point five degrees Celsius.　―熱は（摂氏）37.5度です．

▶ Let me take your blood pressure.　血圧を測りましょう．
— Please hold out your left arm.　―左腕を出して下さい．
— Roll up your sleeve.　―袖をまくって下さい．
— Let me put this cuff on your arm.　―腕にこのカフを巻きましょう．
（機械の場合）
— Please put your arm inside this white cuff.　―この白いカフの中に腕を入れて下さい．
— Relax your arm.　―腕の力を抜いて下さい．
— Your blood pressure is 138 over 85.　―血圧は上が138，下が85です．

▶ I'm going to take your pulse.　脈を測りましょう．
— Please hold out your right hand.　―右手を出して下さい．
— Your pulse is 80 a minute.　―脈は1分間に80です．

ECG / 心電図

▶ I'm going to take an electrocardiogram.　心電図の検査をしましょう．

▶ Please take off your undershirt.　下着のシャツを脱いで下さい．

Lesson 3

▶ **Please take off your socks〔stockings〕, too.**　　靴下〔ストッキング〕も脱いで下さい.

▶ **Please lie on your back on this exam table.**　　この検査台の上に仰向けに寝て下さい.

▶ **Please relax and don't move.**　　楽にして動かないで下さい.

▶ **It'll be over in a few minutes.**　　2，3分で終わります.

▶ **Now, you're finished.**　　さあ，終わりました.

▶ **You can get dressed now.**　　もう服を着てけっこうです.

▶ **Please walk on this treadmill.**　　このトレッドミルの上を歩いて下さい.

▶ **Let me know if you have chest pain or feel pressure or discomfort.**　　胸が痛んだり圧迫感や違和感を覚えたら言って下さい.

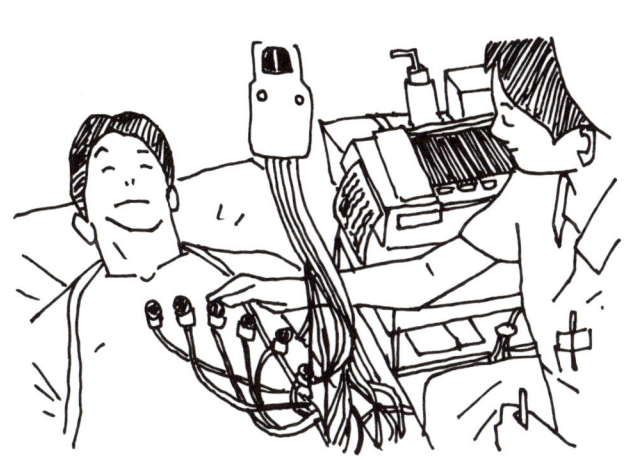

Lesson 4　呼吸器科

A　Cough, Fever, and Headache (Possible disease: acute bronchitis)

○● *Let's Listen!* ●○　　　　　　　　　　　　　　　　　13

■ 状況を思い浮かべながら，CD を聴きましょう．**D/N: Doctor/Nurse　P: Patient**

D/N:　Hello, Ms. Cross. My name is Dr.〔Nurse〕Yagi.
P:　Hello.
D/N:　Please sit down. What can I do for you today?
P:　Well, I've been having these coughs, and I can't sleep at night. I have a headache and a fever as well.
D/N:　I see. How long has this been going on?
P:　Well, about a week ago, I had a cold with a stuffy nose and a sore throat, ...and then, I started coughing. The cough has been going on for about 3 days.
D/N:　What's your cough like?
P:　At first it was dry, and then gradually I started to cough up sputum.
D/N:　Did you take your temperature? How high was it?
P:　It was 38.7℃ this morning.
D/N:　How about your headache?
P:　Well, I have a slight headache ... not severe.
D/N:　Do you get short of breath?
P:　Yes, sometimes I have difficulty breathing.
D/N:　OK, now I'm going to listen to your chest.

A 咳・熱・頭痛（急性気管支炎の疑い）

D/N: 医師/看護師　　P: 患者

D/N: クロスさん，こんにちは．医師〔看護師〕の八木です．
P: こんにちは．
D/N: おかけ下さい．どうなさいましたか．
P: ええ，この咳がずっと続いていて，夜眠れないのです．それに頭が痛く熱もあります．

D/N: わかりました．症状はどのくらい続いているのですか．
P: 1週間ほど前，鼻がつまってのどの痛む風邪をひいたのですが...　それから咳が出始めました．この3日くらいずっと続いているのです．

D/N: どんな咳ですか．
P: 最初は乾いた咳でしたが，だんだん痰がからむようになりました．
D/N: 熱を測りましたか．何度ありましたか．
P: 今朝，（摂氏）38.7度でした．
D/N: 頭痛のほうはどうですか．
P: 少し痛みますが...　ひどくはありません．
D/N: 息切れしますか．
P: はい，時々息苦しくなります．
D/N: それでは，胸の聴診をしましょう．

○● Words and Phrases ●○ 　　　　　　　　　　　　　　　　　　　　　【14】

- [ ] **acute bronchitis** 急性気管支炎
- [ ] **headache** 頭痛
- [ ] **common cold** 感冒
- [ ] **sore throat** のどの痛み
- [ ] **dry** 乾いた
- [ ] **temperature** 体温
- [ ] **breath** 息
- [ ] **have difficulty ...** するのに苦労する
- [ ] **cough** 咳
- [ ] **fever** 発熱
- [ ] **stuffy nose** 鼻づまり
- [ ] **at first** 最初は
- [ ] **sputum** 痰
- [ ] **38.7℃** （摂氏）38.7度
- [ ] **breathe** 息をする

○● Useful Expressions ●○ 　　　　　　　　　　　　　　　　　　　　　【15】

■ 会話モデルの重要表現を確認しましょう．テキストを開いて CD の音声に合わせて発音し，CD のスピードに慣れてきたらテキストを閉じてシャドーイングしてみましょう．

▶ What can I do for you today?	どうなさいましたか．
▶ I see.	わかりました．
▶ How long has this been going on?	症状はどのくらい続いているのですか．
▶ What's your cough like?	どんな咳ですか．
▶ Did you take your temperature?	熱を測りましたか．
▶ How high was it?	何度ありましたか．
▶ How about your headache?	頭痛のほうはどうですか．
▶ Do you get short of breath?	息切れしますか．
▶ OK, now I'm going to listen to your chest.	それでは，胸の聴診をしましょう．

Lesson 4

○● Let's Try! ●○

■ 会話モデルを参考にして，医師・看護師・患者になったつもりで練習して下さい．
■ 咳や痰の性状についてより詳しく問診してみましょう．
　下記の用語ファイルを参考にして下さい．

用語ファイル

■咳の種類

空咳	a dry cough
痰がからむ咳	a productive cough, a cough that brings up sputum
ゼイゼイする咳	a wheezy cough
コンコンする空咳	a hacking cough
犬が吠えるような咳	a barking cough
発作的な咳	a spasmodic cough

■咳の程度

少々の	slight	軽い	mild	中程度の	moderate
ひどい	bad	激しい	severe	ものすごく激しい	violent

■痰の種類

どろどろした痰	thick sputum	さらさらした痰	thin sputum
ねばねばした痰	sticky sputum	泡状の痰	frothy [foamy] sputum
膿のような痰	pus-like sputum	血がにじんだ痰	blood-streaked sputum

■痰の色

透明か白っぽい	clear or white	緑色の	green
黄色味を帯びている	yellowish	ピンク色がかっている	pinkish
赤さび色の	reddish brown	赤い	red
灰色の	gray		

B Physical Examination of the Chest and Back　胸背部の診察

■ 患者さんから正確なデータを得るための具体的な表現を集めました．テキストを開いてCDの音声に合わせて発音し，CDのスピードに慣れてきたらテキストを閉じてシャドーイングをしてみましょう．

▶ I'm going to examine...　　　　　　…を診察しましょう．
　 1. your lungs.　2. your heart.　　　1. 肺　2. 心臓

▶ Please unbutton your shirt〔blouse〕　ワイシャツ〔ブラウス〕のボタンをはずして
　 and pull up your undershirt.　　　下着のシャツを引き上げて下さい．

▶ Let me listen to your lungs and　　肺と心臓の聴診をしましょう．
　 heart.

▶ With your mouth open, please　　　口を開けて普通に息をして下さい．
　 breathe as normal.
— Please breathe in, breathe out, ...in, —息を吸って，吐いて，吸って，吐いて．
　 ...out.
— Again.　　　　　　　　　　　　　—もう一度やって下さい．
— Take a big〔deep〕breath in.　　　　—大きく息を吸って下さい．
— Breathe out as hard and fast as you —できるだけ勢いよく吐いて下さい．
　 can.
— Good, please relax.　　　　　　　　—けっこうです．楽にして下さい．

▶ Let me see your back.　　　　　　　背中を診ましょう．

▶ Please turn around.　　　　　　　　後ろを向いて下さい．
— Say "e."　　　　　　　　　　　　　—「イー」と言ってみて下さい．

▶ I'm going to press〔tap〕your back.　背中を押します〔叩きます〕．

— Does it hurt when I press〔tap〕　　—ここを押す〔叩く〕と痛みますか．
　 here?
— Let me know if you have any pain. —痛いところがあったら言って下さい．

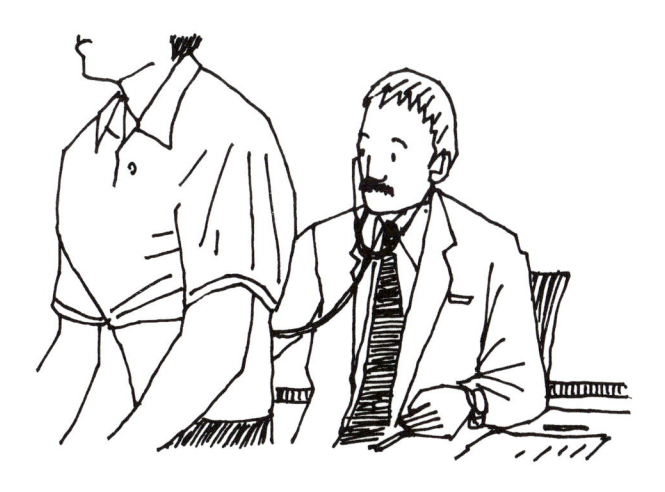

スピーキング攻略のヒント(1)　～英語のリズム～

「聴く力」と「話す力」の両方のカギを握るのは，英語独特のリズムとイントネーションをマスターするか否かにかかっています．英語のリズムは音の強弱の差によって生まれます．「はっきりとやや長めに強く」発音する部分と「速く短めに弱く」発音する部分とに注意を向けて，めりはりをつけて発音します．次の例で確認しましょう．

You're **wél**come.

I'm **sórry** / to have **képt** you / **wáit**ing.

Hów can I / **hélp** you / to**dáy**?

Lesson 5 消化器科

A Abdominal Pain (Possible disease: acute gastritis)

○● Let's Listen! ●○   17

■ 状況を思い浮かべながら，CD を聴きましょう． **D/N: Doctor/Nurse P: Patient**

D/N: Hello, Mr. Hill. I'm Dr.〔Nurse〕Kimura. What can I do for you today?
P: I've got a stomachache.
D/N: When did it start?
P: Several days ago.
D/N: Where exactly is the pain?
P: Here. In the pit of my stomach.
D/N: In what situations do you get it?
P: Well, I get it when I'm hungry.
D/N: What is the pain like? Could you describe it for me?
P: It's heavy, … a dull pain.
D/N: Do you have any other symptoms? Nausea or diarrhea?
P: I've felt nauseous, and I vomited a few times, but I have no diarrhea.
D/N: Have you recently eaten large amounts of spicy food or drunk a large amount of alcohol?
P: I went to a party on the weekend, and I drank enough to get drunk.
D/N: I see. Have you recently taken any medications?
P: No, not particularly.
D/N: Have you ever had a stomach ulcer?
P: No, I haven't.
D: Let me feel your abdomen. Please lie down here, on your back. I think you probably have a stomach upset called acute gastritis.
P: How long will it take to get better?
D: I'll prescribe a medication for your stomach. You'll get better within a few days, but if you don't, make an appointment to see me.
P: All right. Thank you, Doctor.
D: You're welcome.

A 腹痛（急性胃炎の疑い）

D/N: 医師／看護師　　P: 患者

D/N: ヒルさん，こんにちは．医師〔看護師〕の木村です．どうなさいましたか．
P: 　胃が痛んでいるのです．
D/N: 痛み始めたのはいつですか．
P: 　4，5日前からです．
D/N: どこが痛みますか．
P: 　ここ，みぞおちです．
D/N: どんな時に痛みますか．
P: 　そうですね，お腹がすいている時です．
D/N: どんな痛みですか．詳しく話して下さい．
P: 　重苦しくて...鈍い痛みです．
D/N: そのほかの症状がありますか．吐き気は？ 下痢は？
P: 　吐き気がして，2，3回吐きました．でも下痢はしていません．
D/N: 最近，香辛料のきいた物をたくさん食べたり，お酒をかなり飲みましたか．

P: 　週末にパーティがあって，酔っ払うほど飲みました．
D/N: わかりました．最近服用している薬はありますか．
P: 　特にありません．
D/N: これまで胃潰瘍にかかったことがありますか．
P: 　いいえ．ありません．
D: 　お腹を触診しましょう．ここに仰向けに寝て下さい．たぶん急性胃炎でしょう．

P: 　どのくらいでよくなりますか．
D: 　胃薬を処方しましょう．2，3日でよくなりますよ．よくならないようでしたら，診察の予約をして下さい．
P: 　わかりました．ありがとうございます．
D: 　どういたしまして．

● Words and Phrases ●

- [ ] **abdominal pain** 腹痛
- [ ] **stomachache** 胃痛
- [ ] **dull pain** 鈍痛
- [ ] **nausea** 吐き気
- [ ] **diarrhea** 下痢
- [ ] **spicy food** 香辛料のきいた食べ物
- [ ] **recently** 最近
- [ ] **stomach ulcer** 胃潰瘍
- [ ] **make an appointment** 予約する
- [ ] **acute gastritis** 急性胃炎
- [ ] **hungry** 空腹の
- [ ] **symptom** 症状
- [ ] **vomit** 吐く
- [ ] **feel nauseous** 吐き気がする
- [ ] **alcohol** アルコール
- [ ] **abdomen** 腹部
- [ ] **prescribe** 処方する

● Useful Expressions ●

■ 会話モデルの重要表現を確認しましょう．テキストを開いてCDの音声に合わせて発音し，CDのスピードに慣れてきたらテキストを閉じてシャドーイングしてみましょう．

▶ Do you have any other symptoms? Nausea or diarrhea?	そのほかの症状がありますか．吐き気は？下痢は？
▶ Have you recently eaten large amounts of spicy food or drunk a large amount of alcohol?	最近，香辛料のきいた食べ物をたくさん食べたり，お酒をかなり飲みましたか．
▶ Have you recently taken any medications?	最近服用している薬はありますか．
▶ Have you ever had a stomach ulcer?	これまで胃潰瘍にかかったことがありますか．
▶ Let me feel your abdomen.	お腹を触診しましょう．
▶ Please lie down here, on your back.	ここに仰向けに寝て下さい．
▶ I think you probably have a stomach upset called acute gastritis.	たぶん急性胃炎でしょう．

▶ I'll prescribe a medication for your stomach.

胃薬を処方しましょう．

▶ You'll get better within a few days.

2，3日でよくなりますよ．

▶ If you don't, make an appointment to see me.

よくならないようでしたら，診察の予約をして下さい．

▶ You're welcome.

どういたしまして．

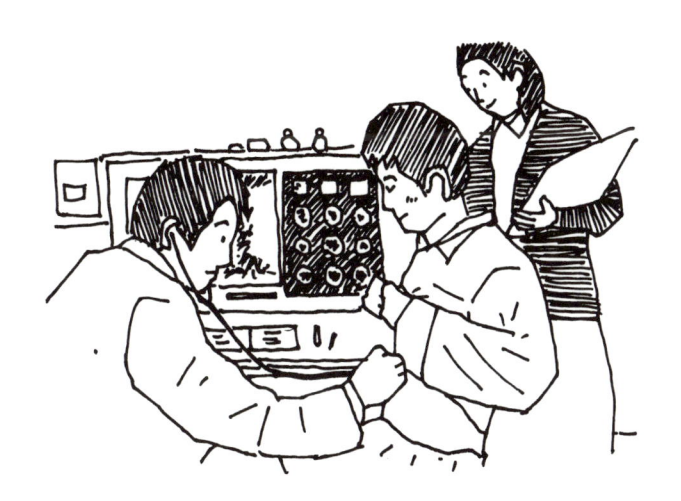

○● Let's Try! ●○

■ 会話モデルを参考にして，医師・看護師・患者になったつもりで練習して下さい．
■ 下痢や便秘など便通に問題のある患者を想定して会話をしてみましょう．
下記の用語ファイルを参考にして下さい．

用語ファイル

■便の形・硬さ　What do your stools look like?
硬い　hard　　軟らかい　soft　　ゆるい　loose　　水のような　watery
泥状の　muddy　　鉛筆状の　pencil-like　　固まっている　well-formed
■便の色　What color are they?
茶色の　brown　　緑がかった　greenish　　黒い　black
タール様　tarry　　白い　white　　赤みがかった　reddish
■便の臭い　What do they smell like?
腐敗臭の　foul-smelling　　酸っぱい臭いの　sour-smelling

B Physical Examination of the Abdomen/Endoscopy 腹部の診察 / 内視鏡検査

■ 患者さんから正確なデータを得るための具体的な表現を集めました．テキストを開いてCDの音声に合わせて発音し，CDのスピードに慣れてきたらテキストを閉じてシャドーイングをしてみましょう． 🎧20

Physical Examination of the Abdomen　腹部の診察

▶ I'm going to examine〔feel〕your abdomen. — お腹を診察〔触診〕しましょう．

▶ Please lie down on your back on the exam table. — 診察台の上に，仰向けに寝て下さい．

▶ Please lower your pants〔skirt〕and show me your abdomen. — ズボン〔スカート〕を下げて，お腹を見せて下さい．

▶ Please pull your knees up and relax your abdomen. — 両膝を立てて，お腹の力を抜いて下さい．

▶ Let me know if you have any pain or lump. — 痛いところやしこりがあったら言って下さい．
— Please point to the place. — —指でさして教えて下さい．
— Does it hurt when I press here? — —ここを押すと痛みますか．
— Does it hurt when I release my hand suddenly? — —手を急に離すと痛みますか．
— Take a big breath in. — —大きく息を吸って下さい．
— Push out your stomach. — —お腹をふくらませて下さい．
— Suck in your stomach. — —お腹をひっこめて下さい．

▶ Please lie on your ... — 今度は…に寝て下さい．
　1. right side.　2. left side. — 1. 右向き　2. 左向き

Endoscopy   内視鏡検査

- ▶ Let me perform an upper endoscopy〔colonoscopy〕.   上部消化管内視鏡〔大腸内視鏡〕検査をしましょう.

- ▶ It'll take about 30 minutes to complete the test.   検査はだいたい30分かかります.

- ▶ Please take off your clothes from the waist up〔from the waist down〕.   上半身〔下半身〕の服を脱いで下さい.

- ▶ Put this gown on.   この検査着を着て下さい.

- ▶ I'm going to give you an injection in the arm.   腕に注射をします.

- ▶ I'm going to anesthetize your throat. Please keep this liquid in your mouth till I say "OK."   のどに麻酔をしますから, 合図するまでこの液体を口の中に含んでおいて下さい.

- ▶ Swallow this tube in one gulp.   管をごくんと飲んで下さい.

- ▶ Try to let your body go limp.   体の力を抜くようにして下さい.

- ▶ I'm going to insert air to expand your digestive tract, so please don't belch〔pass gas〕.   消化管を拡げるために空気を入れますから, しばらくゲップ〔おなら〕を我慢して下さい.

- ▶ Are you all right?   大丈夫ですか.

- ▶ I'm going to perform a biopsy of your stomach〔colon〕to be certain.   念のために胃〔大腸〕の生検をします.

- ▶ Now, you're finished.   さあ, 終わりました.

- ▶ You can get dressed now.   もう服を着てけっこうです.

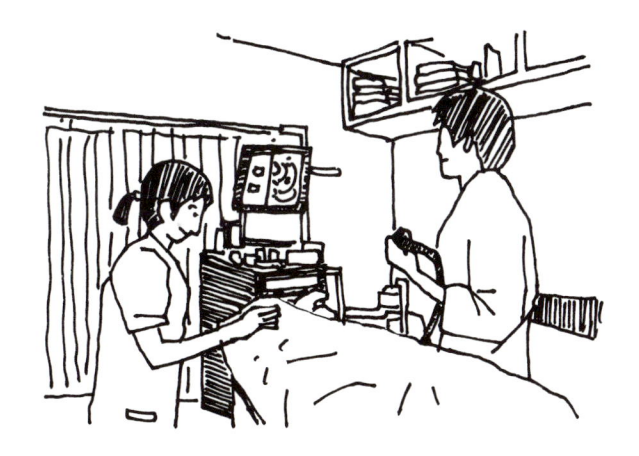

| コラム | 腹痛または胃痛，どっちなの？ |

腹部（横隔膜から骨盤までを含む）をさす医学用語は abdomen で，一般的な語としては stomach が使われる．小児語では tummy を用い，インフォーマルには belly ともいう．
　stomachache は広義には腹痛，狭義には胃痛．そこで a stomachache を訴える患者を診察する医師・看護師は，胃と腸を区別しない腹部全体の痛みとみなし，胃炎から虫垂炎，大腸炎，胆石症，月経困難症にいたるまで，さまざまな疾患を疑うことになる．

Lesson 6 代謝・内分泌科

A Problem Found at the Medical Checkup (Possible disease: diabetes)

○● *Let's Listen!* ●○

■ 状況を思い浮かべながら，CD を聴きましょう．　**D/N: Doctor/Nurse　P: Patient**

D/N: Hello, I'm Dr.〔Nurse〕Tanaka.
P: Hello.
D/N: Are you Ms. Austin?
P: That's right.
D/N: I'm sorry to have kept you waiting. Come and sit down. Well now, how can I help you?
P: I was told at my checkup that my blood sugar level is high.
D/N: Having trouble with a high blood sugar level ... Have you had any symptoms?
P: I feel awfully tired.
D/N: Can you tell me more about that?
P: Well, I've been feeling tired all day long, for no particular reason.
D/N: Have you noticed anything else?
P: I've been putting on weight, gaining more than 5 kilos.
D/N: How is your appetite?
P: Excellent. I feel hungry, and I also get very thirsty.
D/N: Do you pass more urine than usual?
P: Well, yes. I often go to the bathroom.
D/N: Do you have a relative with diabetes?
P: Well, my father has diabetes. Does that mean I will inherit that disease?
D/N: No, but you may have a higher chance of developing the disease than other people. Now then, I'm going to take a blood sample to check your blood sugar level again.

A 健診異常（糖尿病の疑い）

D/N: 医師／看護師　　P: 患者

D/N: こんにちは，医師〔看護師〕の田中です．
P: こんにちは．
D/N: オースティンさんですね．
P: はい，そうです．
D/N: お待たせいたしました．どうぞおかけ下さい．どうなさいましたか．

P: 健診で血糖値が高いと言われました．
D/N: 血糖値が高いのですね．症状はありますか．

P: ええ，ものすごく疲れています．
D/N: そのことについてもっと詳しく話してくれますか．
P: 一日中疲れていて，それも思い当たる理由もないんですけど．
D/N: ほかに何か気がついたことがありますか．
P: 太ってしまって，体重が5キロ以上も増えてしまいました．
D/N: 食欲はどうですか．
P: ええ，すごくあります．お腹がすきますし，それにのどがとても渇くんです．
D/N: いつもより尿が多く出ますか．
P: そうですね．お手洗いにはしょっちゅう行きますけど．
D/N: ご親戚のどなたかに糖尿病の人はいますか．
P: 父がそうですが，それって私にも遺伝するということですか．
D/N: いいえ，ただかかる確率がほかの人より高いと言えるかもしれません．それでは，血液検査をしてもう一度血糖値を調べてみましょう．

○● Words and Phrases ●○

- [ ] **problem** 問題
- [ ] **diabetes** 糖尿病
- [ ] **put on weight** 体重が増える
- [ ] **pass urine** 尿をする
- [ ] **inherit** 遺伝する
- [ ] **blood sample** 血液サンプル
- [ ] **medical checkup** 健診
- [ ] **blood sugar level** 血糖値
- [ ] **feel thirsty** のどが渇く
- [ ] **relative** 親戚
- [ ] **develop the disease** 病気を発症する

○● Useful Expressions ●○

■ 会話モデルの重要表現を確認しましょう．テキストを開いてCDの音声に合わせて発音し，CDのスピードに慣れてきたらテキストを閉じてシャドーイングしてみましょう．

▶ Having trouble with a high blood sugar level ... Have you had any symptoms?	血糖値が高いのですね．症状はありますか．
▶ Can you tell me more about that?	そのことについてもっと詳しく話してくれますか．
▶ Have you noticed anything else?	ほかに何か気がついたことがありますか．
▶ How is your appetite?	食欲はどうですか．
▶ Do you pass more urine than usual?	いつもより尿が多く出ますか．
▶ Do you have a relative with diabetes?	ご親戚のどなたかに糖尿病の人はいますか．
▶ No, but you may have a higher chance of developing the disease than other people.	いいえ，ただかかる確率がほかの人より高いと言えるかもしれません．
▶ Now then, I'm going to take a blood sample to check your blood sugar level again.	それでは，血液検査をしてもう一度血糖値を調べてみましょう．

○● **Let's Try!** ●○

■ 会話モデルを参考にして，医師・看護師・患者になったつもりで練習して下さい．
■ 健診で貧血（anemia）を指摘された患者を想定して会話をしてみましょう．
　下記の用語ファイルを参考にして下さい．

用語ファイル

■貧血の一般的な徴候

顔が青白い	look pale
体が疲れてだるい	feel tired and sluggish
めまいがする	feel dizzy
立ちくらみがする	feel faint
動悸がする	have palpitations
息切れする	get short of breath
ヘモグロビン値が正常より低い	The hemoglobin level is below normal.

B Urine Test and Blood Test　尿検査と血液検査

■ 患者さんから正確なデータを得るための具体的な表現を集めました．テキストを開いてCDの音声に合わせて発音し，CDのスピードに慣れてきたらテキストを閉じてシャドーイングをしてみましょう．

24

Urine Test　尿検査

▶ We need a sample of your urine.　検尿が必要です．

▶ Please use this cup to collect your urine.　このコップに尿をとって下さい．

▶ First, urinate a small amount into the toilet and then fill the cup to about one-third with urine.　まず，トイレに尿を少し出してから，次にコップ3分の1くらいまで入れて下さい．

▶ Please put the cup on this table.　（尿がとれたら）このテーブルの上に置いて下さい．

▶ I'm going to drain the urine from your bladder with this tube.　この管を入れて膀胱から尿をとります．

Blood Test　血液検査

▶ I'm going to take a blood sample.　採血をしましょう．

▶ Please sit down.　お座り下さい．

▶ Please put out your arm and roll up your sleeve.　腕を出して袖をまくって下さい．

— Let me put this tourniquet [tight band] on your arm.　—腕に駆血帯を巻きましょう．

— Please make a fist.　—手を握って下さい．

— Do like this.　—こんなふうに．

— Please relax.　—楽にして下さい．

— Try to let your body go limp.　—体の力を抜くようにして下さい．

Lesson 6

▶ **Have you ever had any allergic reactions to alcohol-based antiseptics, such as reddened skin?**

これまでにアルコール消毒で皮膚が赤くなるなどのアレルギー反応が起こったことはありますか.

▶ **There'll be a little prick.**

ちょっとチクンとしますよ.

▶ **Now, you're finished.**

さあ, 終わりました.

▶ **I'll just put this Band-Aid on your arm, so hold it down for a few minutes.**

このバンドエイドを腕に貼りますから, 2, 3分押さえていて下さい.

▶ **I'm going to prick your ear lobe 〔thumb〕.**

耳〔親指〕から血をとります.

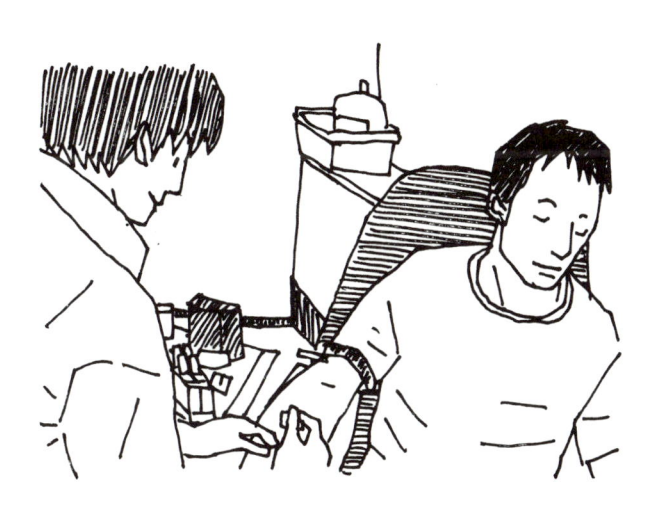

Lesson 7 救急

A Head Injury

○● *Let's Listen!* ●○　　　　　　　　　　　　　　　　25

■ 状況を思い浮かべながら，CD を聴きましょう．　**D/N: Doctor/Nurse　P: Patient**

D/N: Hello, Mr. Smith. Please sit down. I'm Dr.〔Nurse〕Hayashi.
P: Hello.
D/N: Now, what can I do for you today?
P: I've got a bump on the head, and I have a slight pain in my left arm.
D/N: What happened?
P: I fell down in my garden.
D/N: Tell me exactly how it happened.
P: I slipped and fell off a ladder.
D/N: When did it happen?
P: This morning, at about 9 o'clock.
D/N: Then what happened to you?
P: I hit my head against one of the tree stumps.
D/N: Did you lose consciousness?
P: Yes, but only for a while, I think.
D/N: Do you have any other signs or symptoms?
P: Yes, my head aches, but it's not so severe.
D: OK. We'd like to take an X-ray of your arm and a CT of your head. After that I'll take care of your bump.

（検査後に）

D: Judging from the X-ray and CT films, you have nothing to worry about.
P: Good! I'm glad to hear that.
D: If you have any symptoms which cause you concern, come and see me again.

A　頭部外傷

D/N: 医師 / 看護師　　**P:** 患者

D/N: スミスさん，こんにちは．おかけ下さい．医師〔看護師〕の林です．
P: こんにちは．
D/N: どうなさいましたか．
P: 頭にこぶができて，それに左腕が少し痛みます．
D/N: 何があったのですか．
P: 自宅の庭で転倒しました．
D/N: その時の状況を話して下さい．
P: すべってはしごから落ちたのです．
D/N: いつのことですか．
P: 今朝，9時ごろです．
D/N: それで，どうなりましたか．
P: 頭を切り株にぶつけてしまったのです．
D/N: 意識を失いましたか．
P: ええ，でもほんのしばらくだと思います．
D/N: ほかに徴候や症状がありますか．
P: 頭が痛みますが，たいしたことはありません．
D: わかりました．それでは腕のX線写真と頭のCTを撮りましょう．それからこぶの手当てをしましょう．

D: レントゲンとCTから判断すると，心配なことはありません．
P: よかった！　安心しました．
D: 心配な症状が出たらまた受診して下さい．

○● Words and Phrases ●○

- [ ] **head injury** 頭の怪我
- [ ] **happen** 起こる
- [ ] **consciousness** 意識
- [ ] **X-ray** レントゲン
- [ ] **take care of** 手当てする
- [ ] **worry about** 心配する
- [ ] **bump** こぶ
- [ ] **fall off a ladder** はしごから落ちる
- [ ] **ache** 鈍く痛む
- [ ] **CT scan** CT スキャン
- [ ] **judging from** …から判断すると
- [ ] **concern** 心配事

○● Useful Expressions ●○

■ 会話モデルの重要表現を確認しましょう．テキストを開いて CD の音声に合わせて発音し，CD のスピードに慣れてきたらテキストを閉じてシャドーイングしてみましょう．

▶ What happened?	何があったのですか．
▶ Tell me exactly how it happened.	その時の状況を話して下さい．
▶ When did it happen?	いつのことですか．
▶ Then what happened to you?	それで，どうなりましたか．
▶ Did you lose consciousness?	意識を失いましたか．
▶ Do you have any other signs or symptoms?	ほかに徴候や症状がありますか．
▶ OK. We'd like to take an X-ray of your arm and a CT of your head.	わかりました．それでは腕の X 線写真と頭の CT を撮りましょう．
▶ After that I'll take care of your bump.	それからこぶの手当てをしましょう．
▶ Judging from the X-ray and CT films, you have nothing to worry about.	レントゲンと CT から判断すると，心配なことはありません．
▶ If you have any symptoms which cause you concern, come and see me again.	心配な症状が出たらまた受診して下さい．

○● *Let's Try!* ●○

■ 会話モデルを参考にして，医師・看護師・患者になったつもりで練習して下さい．
■ スポーツで怪我をした患者を想定して会話をしてみましょう．
　下記の用語ファイルを参考にして下さい．

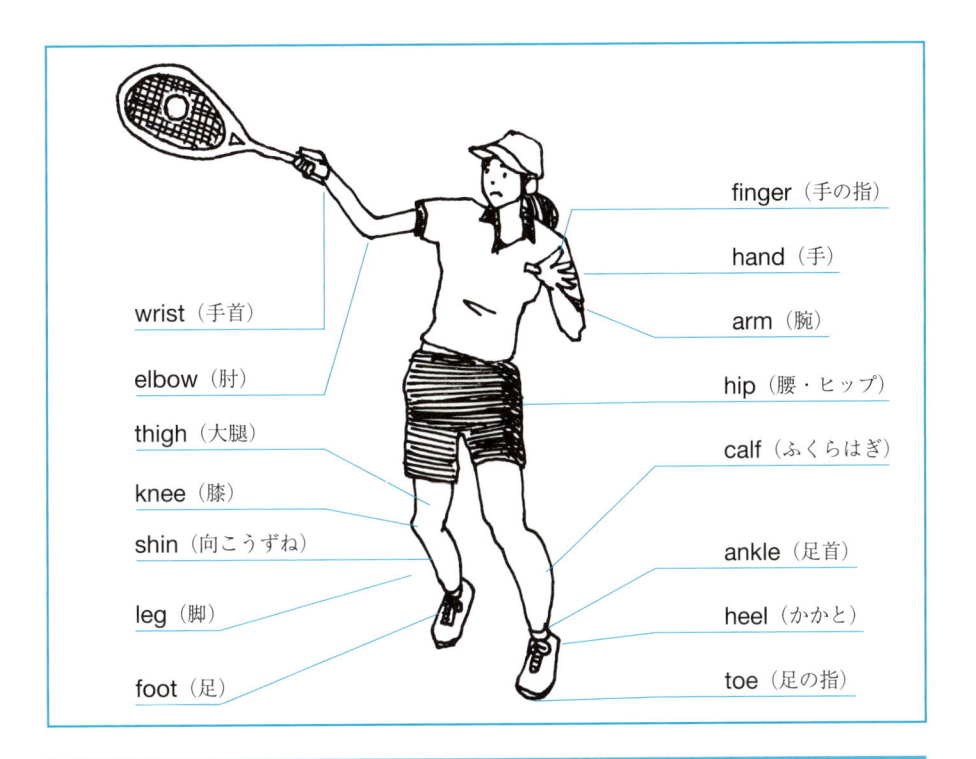

- finger（手の指）
- hand（手）
- arm（腕）
- hip（腰・ヒップ）
- calf（ふくらはぎ）
- ankle（足首）
- heel（かかと）
- toe（足の指）
- wrist（手首）
- elbow（肘）
- thigh（大腿）
- knee（膝）
- shin（向こうずね）
- leg（脚）
- foot（足）

用語ファイル

■手足の怪我

骨折する	break [fracture] a bone
打撲傷を負う	get a bruise
捻挫する	sprain [twist]
アキレス腱を切る	tear the Achilles tendon
肉離れを起こす	have a torn muscle
足がつる	have a leg cramp
脱臼する	dislocate
突き指する	sprain a finger

B X-ray, CT, and MRI　　X線検査とCT・MRI検査

■ 患者さんから正確なデータを得るための具体的な表現を集めました．テキストを開いてCDの音声に合わせて発音し，CDのスピードに慣れてきたらテキストを閉じてシャドーイングをしてみましょう．

🎧 28

X-ray　　　　　　　　　　　　　　　　X線検査

▶ I'm going to take an X-ray of your...　　…のレントゲンを撮りましょう．
　1. chest.　2. abdomen.　3. cervical 　　1. 胸部　2. 腹部　3. 頸椎〔首〕　4. 腰椎
　spine〔neck〕.　4. lumbar spine.　　　　5. 胃
　5. stomach.

▶ Please take off your clothes from　　上半身の服を脱いで下さい．
　the waist up.

▶ Remove all of your jewelry as well.　　装飾品もぜんぶ取って下さい．

▶ Put this gown on.　　この検査着を着て下さい．

▶ Please stand with your head facing　　前を向いて立って下さい．
　forward.

▶ Put your arms by your side, like　　手を横に置いて下さい，こんなふうに．
　this.

▶ Take a big breath in and hold.　　大きく息を吸って，止めて下さい．

▶ Relax, please.　　楽にして下さい．

▶ Stand sideways, this time.　　今度は，横を向いて下さい．

▶ Please swallow this special drink　　この液〔バリウム〕を飲んで下さい．
　〔barium mixture〕.

▶ Empty the cup in one gulp.　　コップの中身を一気に飲んで下さい．

▶ Hold on without belching.　　ゲップをしないで我慢して下さい．

▶ Lie down on this exam table.	この検査台の上に横になって下さい．
▶ The table will move you into different positions.	台はいろいろな方向に動きます．
▶ You may feel some pressure.	少し圧迫される感じがするかもしれません．
▶ Let me know when it hurts.	痛かったらおっしゃって下さい．
▶ Now, you're finished.	さあ，終わりました．
▶ You can get dressed now.	もう服を着てけっこうです．
▶ Please drink plenty of fluids to prevent getting constipated.	便秘をしないように，水分をたくさんとって下さい．
▶ It may be helpful to take a laxative.	下剤を飲んでもいいですよ．

CT/MRI　　　　　　　　　　　　CT/MRI

▶ I'm going to [Let me] take a CT scan [an MRI] of your... 1. head.　2. chest.　3. heart.　4. abdomen.	…のCT〔MRI〕検査をしましょう． 1. 頭部　2. 胸部　3. 心臓　4. 腹部
▶ It'll take a few [30] minutes or so to complete the test.	検査はだいたい2，3分〔30分〕かかります．
▶ The test is painless, so don't worry.	検査は痛くありませんから心配しないで下さい．
▶ Have you ever had any allergic reactions to a contrast medium?	これまでに造影剤でアレルギー反応を起こしたことはありますか．
▶ Have you had any metal implants inserted in your body, such as a pacemaker, clips, or artificial joints?	これまでにペースメーカー，クリップ，人工関節などの金属を体内に埋め込む手術をしたことがありますか．

▶ Please remove all metallic objects, such as glasses, watch, jewelry, bobby pins, dentures, and others.	眼鏡，時計，装飾品，ヘアピン，入れ歯などすべての金属製品をとって下さい．
▶ Please take off your clothes from the waist up.	上半身の服を脱いで下さい．
▶ Put this gown on.	この検査着を着て下さい．
▶ I'm going to give you a contrast medium to highlight the area to be examined.	検査部位をはっきりさせるために造影剤を投与します．
▶ Please lie on your back on this exam table.	この検査台の上に仰向けに寝て下さい．
▶ I'll set up this equipment for you. It won't hurt you.	この器具をつけますが，痛くありませんから．
▶ Please try to relax and don't move.	楽にして動かないで下さい．
▶ Keep still until the test is finished.	検査が済むまでじっとしていて下さい．
▶ You can listen to music during the test, so try to relax.	検査の間，音楽を聴いて楽にしていて下さい．
▶ The machine makes a whirring〔knocking〕noise, but don't worry.	検査中，機械がブーン〔カチカチ〕という音を出しますが，心配いりません．
▶ The table will be moving slowly.	台がゆっくり動いていきます．
▶ Please take a big breath in. — Hold. — Relax.	大きく息を吸って下さい． ―息を止めて下さい． ―楽にして下さい．
▶ Now, you're finished.	さあ，終わりました．
▶ You can get dressed now.	もう服を着てけっこうです．

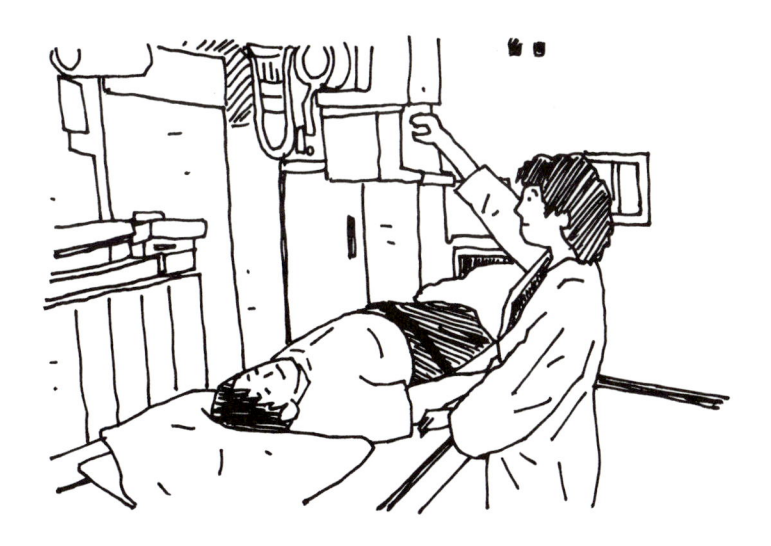

スピーキング攻略のヒント(2)　〜イントネーション(声の抑揚)〜

文の最後を上り調子で言うか，それとも下り調子で言うかに注意しましょう．

a) 質問するときには上昇調で発音します．
   Can you tell me a little about yourself ? (↗)

b) 疑問詞を使う文は原則として下り調子で発音しますが，上昇調で発音すると，相手に好意をもっているというやさしい印象を与えます．以下の文を比べて下さい．
   What's your name, please ? (↗)…「お名前を言って下さい」
   What's your name, please ? (↘)…「名前を言いなさい」という詰問調．

c) 会話では，形式は疑問文ではなくても，疑問符をつけて上昇調で発音することがあります．意味が異なるときがあるので，注意して下さい．
   Oh, you have a severe headache ? (↗)…「ひどい頭痛があるのですか」
   I beg your pardon ? (↗)…「もう一度言って下さい」
   I beg your pardon. (↘)…「ごめんなさい」という謝罪．

d) 長い文では，ことばが続くことを知らせる合図として，軽い上昇調で発音します．
   First, urinate a small amount into the toilet (↗) **and then fill the cup to about one-third with urine.**

Lesson 8 泌尿器科

A Back Pain and Bloody Urine (Possible disease: kidney stones)

○● **Let's Listen!** ●○ **29**

■ 状況を思い浮かべながら，CD を聴きましょう。 D/N: Doctor/Nurse　P: Patient

D/N: Good morning. I'm Dr.〔Nurse〕Okada.
P: Good morning.
D/N: Mr. Locke?
P: That's right.
D/N: Please sit down. Now, what can I do for you today?
P: I've got a pain in my back.
D/N: Where does it hurt?
P: It's in my right side.
D/N: Could you point to where the pain is?
P: Around here.
D/N: What is the pain like? Could you describe it for me?
P: It's a griping pain, really intense.
D/N: Have you ever had this kind of pain before?
P: Yes, two weeks ago. Then it went away after a while.
D/N: I see. Have you noticed anything else?
P: I feel nauseous, and I get cold sweats, too.
D/N: Any problems urinating?
P: No, but my urine is cloudy and appears slightly reddish.
D/N: Have you ever had gout?
P: Yes, several years ago. But I have no problem now.
D/N: Have you been told at a checkup that your uric acid level is high?
P: Well, I haven't had any checkup since I came to Japan two years ago.
　　　………
D: I think you probably have kidney stones. We need to run some tests for an accurate diagnosis, such as a blood test and a urine test. And then, let's do an X-ray and an ultrasound test.

A 背部痛・血尿（腎結石の疑い）

D/N: 医師 / 看護師　P: 患者

D/N: おはようございます．医師〔看護師〕の岡田です．
P: おはようございます．
D/N: ロックさんですね．
P: はい，そうです．
D/N: どうぞおかけ下さい．どうなさいましたか．
P: 背中が痛むのです．
D/N: どこが痛みますか．
P: 右のわき腹です．
D/N: 痛む場所を指でさして教えて下さい．
P: このあたりです．
D/N: どんな痛みですか．詳しく話して下さい．
P: 差し込むような，すごく激しい痛みです．
D/N: 以前，このような痛みがありましたか．
P: ええ，2週間前に．その時はしばらくしたら治まりました．
D/N: わかりました．ほかに何か気になることがありますか．
P: 吐き気がして，それに冷や汗も出ます．
D/N: 排尿に問題がありますか．
P: いいえ，でも尿は濁っていて，少し赤みがかっているように見えます．
D/N: 痛風の既往はありますか．
P: ええ，数年前に．でも今は問題ありません．
D/N: 健診で尿酸値が高いと言われましたか．
P: ええと，健診は2年前日本に来てから受けていません．
　　　　………
D: 腎結石の疑いがあります．正確に診断するために血液検査，尿検査などが必要です．それからX線，超音波の検査をしましょう．

● Words and Phrases ●

- [ ] **kidney stone** 腎結石
- [ ] **bloody urine** 血尿
- [ ] **griping pain** 差し込むような痛み
- [ ] **cold sweats** 冷や汗
- [ ] **cloudy** 濁った
- [ ] **uric acid** 尿酸
- [ ] **ultrasound test** 超音波検査
- [ ] **back pain** 背部痛
- [ ] **hurt** 痛む
- [ ] **intense** 激しい
- [ ] **urinate** 尿をする
- [ ] **gout** 痛風
- [ ] **accurate diagnosis** 正確な診断

● Useful Expressions ●

■ 会話モデルの重要表現を確認しましょう．テキストを開いて CD の音声に合わせて発音し，CD のスピードに慣れてきたらテキストを閉じてシャドーイングしてみましょう．

▶ Where does it hurt?	どこが痛みますか．
▶ Could you point to where the pain is?	痛む場所を指でさして教えて下さい．
▶ Any problems urinating?	排尿に問題がありますか．
▶ Have you ever had gout?	痛風の既往はありますか．
▶ Have you been told at a checkup that your uric acid level is high?	健診で尿酸値が高いと言われましたか．
▶ I think you probably have kidney stones.	腎結石の疑いがあります．
▶ We need to run some tests for an accurate diagnosis, such as a blood test and a urine test.	正確に診断するために血液検査，尿検査などが必要です．
▶ And then, let's do an X-ray and an ultrasound test.	それから X 線，超音波の検査をしましょう．

○● **Let's Try!** ●○

■ 会話モデルを参考にして，医師・看護師・患者になったつもりで練習して下さい．
■ 膀胱炎（bladder infection [cystitis]）の症状を訴える患者を想定して会話をしてみましょう．
　下記の用語ファイルを参考にして下さい．

用語ファイル

■膀胱炎の一般的な症状

排尿時に焼け付くような痛みがある	have a burning pain when urinating
いつもより尿の回数が多い	urinate more often than usual
残尿感がある	feel that the bladder is not empty after urination
尿は濁っている	have cloudy urine
尿意を突然催す	have a sudden need to urinate

B Ultrasound Test　　超音波検査（エコー）

■ 患者さんから正確なデータを得るための具体的な表現を集めました．テキストを開いてCDの音声に合わせて発音し，CDのスピードに慣れてきたらテキストを閉じてシャドーイングをしてみましょう．

▶ I'm going to do the ultrasound on your...
1. abdomen.　2. thyroid.
3. breasts.　4. heart.

…の超音波検査をしましょう．
1. 腹部　2. 甲状腺
3. 乳房　4. 心臓

▶ Please take off your clothes from the waist up.

上半身の服を脱いで下さい．

▶ Please lie on your back on the exam table.

検査台の上に仰向けに寝て下さい．

▶ Please roll your skirt〔pants〕down from your abdomen.

スカート〔ズボン〕をさげてお腹を出して下さい．

▶ You may feel a little gentle pressure, but it is not painful.

多少押される感じがしますが，痛くはありません．

▶ Please...
1. inflate〔push out〕your stomach.
2. suck in your stomach.
3. breathe as normal.
4. take a big breath in.
5. hold.
6. relax.

どうぞ…
1. お腹をふくらませて下さい．
2. お腹をひっこめて下さい．
3. 普通に息をして下さい．
4. 大きく息を吸って下さい．
5. 息を止めて下さい．
6. 楽にして下さい．

▶ Please lie on your right〔left〕side.

右向き〔左向き〕に寝て下さい．

▶ Please lie on your stomach.

腹ばいに寝て下さい．

▶ Now, you're finished.

さあ，終わりました．

▶ You can get dressed now.

もう服を着てけっこうです．

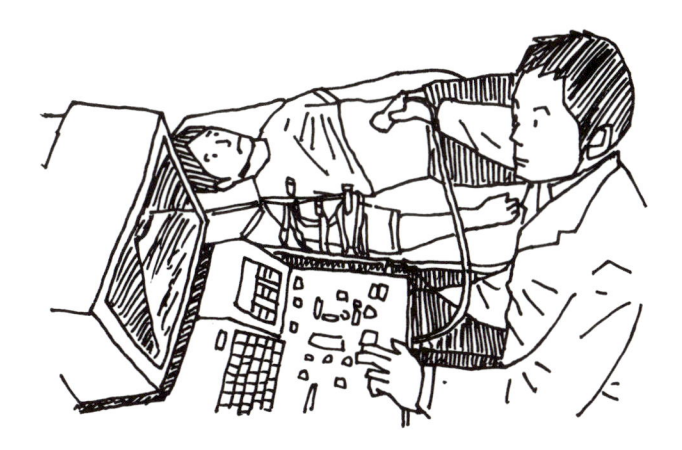

スピーキング攻略のヒント(3)　〜音の連結〜

自然な話ことばの中では，音と音がつながる現象がよく起こります．次の例をCDで確認しましょう．

Please fill out this form. (p. 2)

How can I help you today? (p. 8)

Have you ever had a stomach ulcer? (p. 26)

Come and sit down. (p. 34)

Is there anyone with you today whom you'd like to have join us? (p. 54)

Lesson 9 乳腺外科

A Lump in the Breast (Possible disease: breast cancer)

○● *Let's Listen!* ●○　　　　　　　　　　　　　　　33

■ 状況を思い浮かべながら，CD を聴きましょう． **D: Doctor　P: Patient**

D: Hello, I'm Dr. Katoh. Are you Ms. Neal?
P: That's right.
D: I'm sorry to have kept you waiting. Well now, how can I help you?
P: I noticed a lump in my right breast a week ago.
D: Do you have any other symptoms? Any pain or nipple discharge?
P: No, I don't.
D: When was your last period?
P: It started August 16th and lasted about a week.
D: Has anyone in your immediate family had breast cancer?
P: No.
D: Have you ever had a mammography?
P: Yes, I had one last fall.
D: Have you been doing regular breast self-exams?
P: Yes, and I noticed the lump while I was taking a bath.
D: Now, I'm going to examine your breast. Please take off your clothes from the waist up and lie down on the exam table, on your back.

（診察と検査後に）

D: Let me explain the results of the tests. Is there anyone with you today whom you'd like to have join us?
P: My husband is in the waiting room. Is it all right if he joins us?
D: Certainly.
D: I'm sorry, but judging from the breast examination and the mammography, I think you probably have breast cancer.
P: Really?
D: You need to have more thorough examinations for an accurate diagnosis. I'm going to refer you to a breast specialist for consultation.

A 乳房のしこり（乳癌の疑い）

D: 医師　P: 患者

D: こんにちは，医師の加藤です．ニールさんですね．
P: はい，そうです．
D: お待たせいたしました．どうなさいましたか．
P: 1週間ほど前に右乳房のしこりに気づきました．
D: そのほかの症状がありますか．痛みや乳首からの分泌物がありますか．
P: ありません．
D: 最終月経はいつでしたか．
P: 8月16日から1週間ほどです．
D: 血のつながったご家族に乳癌の人がいますか．
P: いいえ．
D: 以前マンモグラフィを受けたことがありますか．
P: はい，昨年の秋に受けました．
D: これまで乳房自己触診を定期的にしていましたか．
P: はい，入浴中しこりに気がついたのです．
D: それでは乳房の診察をしましょう．服は上半身脱いで，診察台の上に仰向けに寝て下さい．

D: それでは検査結果についてお話しましょう．今日一緒に話を聞いてもらいたい人は来ていますか．
P: 夫が待ち合室にいますので，一緒に話を聞いてもよいですか．
D: もちろんいいですよ．
D: 残念ながら，触診とマンモグラフィ検査から判断すると，乳癌の疑いがあります．

P: 本当ですか．
D: 正確な診断をするためには，精密検査をする必要があります．乳癌の専門医をご紹介しましょう．

○● Words and Phrases ●○

- [ ] **lump** しこり
- [ ] **nipple discharge** 乳首からの分泌物
- [ ] **mammography** マンモグラフィ
- [ ] **take off clothes** 服を脱ぐ
- [ ] **certainly** もちろん
- [ ] **breast specialist** 乳癌専門医
- [ ] **breast** 乳房
- [ ] **period** 月経
- [ ] **breast self-exam** 乳房自己触診
- [ ] **result** 結果
- [ ] **thorough examination** 精密検査
- [ ] **consultation** 受診,相談

○● Useful Expressions ●○

■ 会話モデルの重要表現を確認しましょう．テキストを開いて CD の音声に合わせて発音し，CD のスピードに慣れてきたらテキストを閉じてシャドーイングしてみましょう．

▶ Any pain or nipple discharge?	痛みや乳首からの分泌物がありますか．
▶ When was your last period?	最終月経はいつでしたか．
▶ Has anyone in your immediate family had breast cancer?	血のつながったご家族に乳癌の人がいますか．
▶ Have you ever had a mammography?	以前マンモグラフィを受けたことがありますか．
▶ Have you been doing regular breast self-exams?	これまで乳房自己触診を定期的にしていましたか．
▶ Now, I'm going to examine your breast.	それでは乳房の診察をしましょう．
▶ Please take off your clothes from the waist up and lie down on the exam table, on your back.	服は上半身脱いで，診察台の上に仰向けに寝て下さい．
▶ Let me explain the results of the tests.	それでは検査結果についてお話しましょう．
▶ Is there anyone with you today whom you'd like to have join us?	今日一緒に話を聞いてもらいたい人は来ていますか．

▶ **Certainly.**   もちろんいいですよ．

▶ **I'm sorry, but judging from the breast examination and the mammography, I think you probably have breast cancer.**   残念ながら，触診とマンモグラフィ検査から判断すると，乳癌の疑いがあります．

▶ **You need to have more thorough examinations for an accurate diagnosis.**   正確な診断をするためには，精密検査をする必要があります．

▶ **I'm going to refer you to a breast specialist for consultation.**   乳癌の専門医をご紹介しましょう．

○● *Let's Try!* ●○

■ 会話モデルを参考にして，医師・患者になったつもりで練習して下さい．
■ 月経についてより詳しく問診してみましょう．
　下記の用語ファイルを参考にして下さい．

用語ファイル	
■月経についての情報	
初経年齢はいつか	How old were you when you had your first period?
最終月経はいつか	When was your last period?
月経周期はどのくらいか	How many days usually pass between your periods?
月経に規則性はあるか	Are your periods regular or irregular?
月経期間はどのくらいか	How many days do your periods last?
出血量はどうか	What is your usual flow?
少なめ	light
ふつう	normal
多め	heavy
月経痛はどうか	Do you have any pain or discomfort during your periods?

B Surgical Consultation　　手術の説明

■ 患者さんから正確なデータを得るための具体的な表現を集めました．テキストを開いてCDの音声に合わせて発音し，CDのスピードに慣れてきたらテキストを閉じてシャドーイングをしてみましょう．

▶ The surgery you're going to have is...　　手術は…を予定しています．
  1. cataract surgery.　　1. 白内障手術
  2. a coronary artery bypass.　　2. 冠動脈バイパス術
  3. an appendectomy.　　3. 虫垂切除術
  4. breast-conserving surgery.　　4. 乳房温存術

▶ I need your consent to do this surgery.　　この手術を行うためにあなたの同意が必要です．

▶ Please read this (informed) consent form carefully and sign it.　　この同意書をよく読んで，サインして下さい．
— Do you have anyone who can sign it for you?　　—どなたかサインしてくれる人はいますか．

▶ Your surgery is scheduled for Wednesday morning.　　水曜日午前に手術の予定です．

▶ You have to stay in the hospital for about 10 days.　　10日間ほどの入院が必要です．

▶ Your anesthesiologist is going to give you the details of the anesthesia later.　　麻酔については，後で麻酔医から詳しく説明があります．

▶ (Do you have) any questions?　　ご質問がありますか．

Lesson 10 脳神経科

A Dizziness (Possible disease: intracerebral hemorrhage)

○● *Let's Listen!* ●○ 　　　　　　　　　　　　　　　　　　　37

■ 状況を思い浮かべながら，CD を聴きましょう． **D/N: Doctor/Nurse　P: Patient**

D/N: Hello, I'm Dr.〔Nurse〕Sano. It's Mr. Glass, isn't it?
P: That's right.
D/N: What can I do for you today?
P: I've been feeling dizzy since this morning.
D/N: What's the dizziness like? Can you describe it for me?
P: I feel lightheaded.
D/N: When and in what situation did it come on?
P: About 3 hours ago. I was working, and then it came on suddenly when I was going to the bathroom.
D/N: How was it then? Mild or severe?
P: Pretty severe. It was difficult to stand up and walk. But it got much better after an hour or so.
D/N: When you are standing still, do you feel unsteady?
P: Yes, and I have difficulty walking.
D/N: Do you find it difficult to balance yourself?
P: Yes, I do. I stagger and can't walk straight.
D/N: Have you ever had this dizziness before?
P: No, it's the first time.
D/N: Do you have any other symptoms? Any double vision?
P: No.
D/N: How about numbness, tingling, or weakness in any part of your body?
P: No problem there.
D: OK, I'm going to take a CT scan〔an MRI〕of your head.

（CT 検査後に）

D: The result of the CT shows that there's some slight bleeding. You need to be admitted to the hospital.

A　めまい（脳出血の疑い）

D/N: 医師／看護師　**P:** 患者

- **D/N:** こんにちは．医師〔看護師〕の佐野です．グラスさんですね．
- **P:** そうです．
- **D/N:** 今日はどうなさいましたか．
- **P:** 今朝からずっとめまいがしているんです．
- **D/N:** どんなめまいですか．詳しく話して下さい．
- **P:** 頭がふわっとした感じです．
- **D/N:** いつどんなときに起こったのですか．
- **P:** 3時間くらい前です．仕事中，トイレに立ったとき突然起こりました．

- **D/N:** そのときめまいの程度はどうでしたか．軽かったですか，激しかったですか．
- **P:** とてもひどくて，立ったり歩いたりできないほどでした．でも1，2時間したらだいぶよくなりました．
- **D/N:** じっと立っているときふらつきますか．
- **P:** ええ，それに歩きにくいです．
- **D/N:** バランスをとるのが難しいのですか．
- **P:** そうなんです．よろけて真っ直ぐ歩けません．
- **D/N:** 以前にこのようなめまいが起こったことがありますか．
- **P:** いいえ，今回が初めてです．
- **D/N:** ほかに何か症状がありますか．物が二重に見えることは？
- **P:** いいえ．
- **D/N:** 体の一部がしびれたり，チクチクしたり，力が入らないなどの症状がありますか．
- **P:** いいえ，それは問題ありません．
- **D:** それでは，頭部のCT〔MRI〕をとりましょう．

- **D:** CTの結果では少し出血がみられます．入院が必要です．

○● Words and Phrases ●○

- [ ] **intracerebral hemorrhage** 脳出血
- [ ] **stand still** じっと立っている
- [ ] **balance** バランスをとる
- [ ] **walk straight** 真っ直ぐ歩く
- [ ] **numbness** しびれ
- [ ] **weakness** 脱力
- [ ] **be admitted to the hospital** 入院する
- [ ] **feel lightheaded** 頭がふわっとする
- [ ] **feel unsteady** ふらつく
- [ ] **stagger** よろける
- [ ] **vision** 視野
- [ ] **tingling** チクチク感
- [ ] **bleeding** 出血

○● Useful Expressions ●○

■ 会話モデルの重要表現を確認しましょう．テキストを開いてCDの音声に合わせて発音し，CDのスピードに慣れてきたらテキストを閉じてシャドーイングしてみましょう．

▶ What's the dizziness like? Can you describe it for me?	どんなめまいですか．詳しく話して下さい．
▶ When and in what situation did it come on?	いつどんなときに起こったのですか．
▶ How was it then? Mild or severe?	そのときめまいの程度はどうでしたか．軽かったですか，激しかったですか．
▶ When you are standing still, do you feel unsteady?	じっと立っているときふらつきますか．
▶ Do you find it difficult to balance yourself?	バランスをとるのが難しいのですか．
▶ Have you ever had this dizziness before?	以前にこのようなめまいが起こったことがありますか．
▶ Do you have any other symptoms?	ほかに何か症状がありますか．
▶ Any double vision?	物が二重に見えることは？
▶ How about numbness, tingling, or weakness in any part of your body?	体の一部がしびれたり，チクチクしたり，力が入らないなどの症状がありますか．

▶ OK, I'm going to take a CT scan 〔an MRI〕of your head.　　それでは，頭部のCT〔MRI〕をとりましょう．

▶ The result of the CT shows that there's some slight bleeding.　　CTの結果では少し出血がみられます．

▶ You need to be admitted to the hospital.　　入院が必要です．

○● ***Let's Try!*** ●○

■ 会話モデルを参考にして，医師・看護師・患者になったつもりで練習して下さい．
■ メニエール病(Ménière's disease)の症状を訴える患者を想定して会話をしてみましょう．下記の用語ファイルを参考にして下さい．

用語ファイル

■メニエール病の一般的な症状

めまいの発作を繰り返す	have attacks of dizziness repeatedly
突然あらゆる物がぐるぐる回る	everything seems to spin around suddenly
吐き気がする	feel nauseous
嘔吐する	vomit
耳がふさがった感じがする	feel as if the ears are blocked up
耳がよく聞こえない	have difficulty hearing
耳鳴りがする	have a ringing in the ears

B Hospital Admission   入院

■ 患者さんから正確なデータを得るための具体的な表現を集めました．テキストを開いてCDの音声に合わせて発音し，CDのスピードに慣れてきたらテキストを閉じてシャドーイングをしてみましょう． 🎧40

Before Admission	入院前

▶ Please make an appointment for hospitalization at the admitting office.　　入院受付係で入院の予約をして下さい．

▶ Please read this brochure on admission.　　この入院説明書をお読み下さい．

— You will find information about what to bring, visiting hours, and so on.　　—持ってくるもの，面会時間などの説明がのっています．

▶ If you have someone who could interpret for you, please write down his〔her〕name and telephone number.　　通訳をしてくれる人がいたら，お名前と電話番号を書いて下さい．

▶ Please write your emergency contact number.　　緊急連絡先を書いて下さい．

▶ Please bring any medications you are taking.　　現在飲んでいる薬をお持ち下さい．

▶ Please do not bring valuables, other than a small amount of money, to the hospital.　　小額のお金のほか貴重品は持ってこないで下さい．

▶ Having someone stay with you isn't necessary〔is necessary〕in this hospital.　　当病院では付き添いは必要ありません〔必要です〕．

▶ If you have any other questions about your admission, please ask the admitting office.　　その他，入院についてご質問がありましたら，入院受付係にお尋ね下さい．

On the Day of Admission　　入院当日

▶ Hello, Mr.〔Mrs./Ms./Miss〕Cross.　　こんにちは，クロスさん．

▶ My name is Ms. Nakamura〔Dr. Nakamura〕. I'm your nurse〔doctor〕.　　担当看護師〔担当医〕の中村です．

▶ You'll be in room 325.　　あなたの病室は 325 号室です．

▶ I'll show you your room〔the floor〕.　　それでは病室〔病棟〕をご案内しましょう．

▶ Please change into your pajamas.　　寝間着に着替えて下さい．

▶ Here's your identification band. Let me attach it to your wrist.　　これはあなたの ID バンドです．手首につけましょう．
— Please don't remove it during your stay.　　―入院中はずさないで下さい．

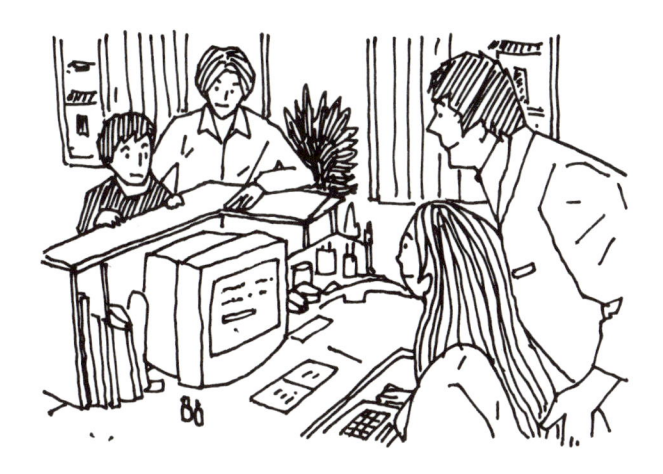

スピーキング攻略のヒント(4)　～音の脱落～

自然な話ことばの中では，語と語の間で隣り合う音のどちらかが脱落することがよくあります．次の例をCDで確認しましょう．

Goo<u>d</u> mornin<u>g</u>.（p. 2）

Are you all righ<u>t</u>?（p. 32）

Have you notice<u>d</u> anything else?（p. 48）

Your nex<u>t</u> checkup is February 3rd, Wednesday.（p. 83）

Lesson 11 心療内科・精神科

A Fatigue, Loss of Weight, and Sleep Disorder (Possible disease: adjustment disorder)

○● *Let's Listen!* ●○   41

■ 状況を思い浮かべながら，CD を聴きましょう。 D/N: Doctor/Nurse   P: Patient

D/N: Hello, Come on in and sit down, please. I'm Dr.〔Nurse〕Shoji. Well, Mr. Brown, what can I do for you today?
P: I'm losing weight, and I feel tired all the time.
D/N: How much weight have you lost?
P: About 5 kilograms. Now I weigh 65 kilograms.
D/N: Do you have any problems sleeping?
P: Yes, I have difficulty falling asleep, and I wake up in the middle of the night.
D/N: How long have you noticed these problems?
P: Almost six months.
D/N: Anything else apart from these problems? Any fever?
P: No.
D/N: How about your appetite? Has it changed at all?
P: Well, it's rather poor.
D/N: Do you feel nauseous?
P: No, I'm OK.
D/N: How are your bowel movements?
P: Oh, they're regular.
D/N: Do you have any pain in your stomach or abdomen?
P: Now that you mention it, my food often feels heavy on my stomach.
D/N: How long have you been in Japan?
P: About a year.
D/N: Has your life changed recently?
P: Yes. I was assigned to a new position in my company six months ago.
D/N: Are you busy with your work?
P: Yes. I'm often up all night working.
D/N: OK, now let's do your physical exam.

A 疲労・体重減少・睡眠障害（適応障害の疑い）

D/N: 医師／看護師　**P:** 患者

- **D/N:** こんにちは．入っておかけ下さい．医師〔看護師〕の庄司です．ブラウンさん，どうなさいましたか．
- **P:** 体重が減ってきて，ずっと体がだるいのです．
- **D/N:** 体重はどのくらい減りましたか．
- **P:** 約5キロです．現在は65キロです．
- **D/N:** 睡眠に何か問題がありますか．
- **P:** ええ，寝つきが悪くて，夜中に目が覚めてしまうのです．
- **D/N:** その症状はどのくらい続いていますか．
- **P:** ほとんど6か月になります．
- **D/N:** そのほかに何か症状がありますか．熱は？
- **P:** ありません．
- **D/N:** 食欲はどうですか．変化がありましたか．
- **P:** そうですね，食欲はあまりありません．
- **D/N:** 吐き気はありますか．
- **P:** それは，だいじょうぶです．
- **D/N:** 便通はどうですか．
- **P:** 規則的にあります．
- **D/N:** 腹痛はありますか．
- **P:** そう言えば，最近，胃がもたれることが多いような気がします．
- **D/N:** 日本に来てどのくらいになりますか．
- **P:** 約1年です．
- **D/N:** 最近，生活に変化はありましたか．
- **P:** ちょうど半年前から新しい職場に配置換えになりました．
- **D/N:** 仕事は忙しいですか．
- **P:** ええ．徹夜で仕事をすることも多いです．
- **D/N:** それでは，診察しましょう．

○● Words and Phrases ●○ 〔42〕

- [ ] fatigue 疲労
- [ ] adjustment disorder 適応障害
- [ ] fall asleep 寝入る
- [ ] apart from ... 以外は
- [ ] loss of weight 体重減少
- [ ] weigh 体重が...ある
- [ ] wake up 目覚める
- [ ] bowel movement 便通

○● Useful Expressions ●○ 〔43〕

■ 会話モデルの重要表現を確認しましょう．テキストを開いて CD の音声に合わせて発音し，CD のスピードに慣れてきたらテキストを閉じてシャドーイングしてみましょう．

▶ How much weight have you lost?	体重はどのくらい減りましたか．
▶ Do you have any problems sleeping?	睡眠に何か問題がありますか．
▶ How long have you noticed these problems?	その症状はどのくらい続いていますか．
▶ Anything else apart from these problems? Any fever?	そのほかに何か症状がありますか．熱は？
▶ How about your appetite? Has it changed at all?	食欲はどうですか．変化がありましたか．
▶ Do you feel nauseous?	吐き気はありますか．
▶ How are your bowel movements?	便通はどうですか．
▶ Do you have any pain in your stomach or abdomen?	腹痛はありますか．
▶ How long have you been in Japan?	日本に来てどのくらいになりますか．
▶ Has your life changed recently?	最近，生活に変化はありましたか．
▶ Are you busy with your work?	仕事は忙しいですか．

○● *Let's Try!* ●○

■ 会話モデルを参考にして，医師・看護師・患者になったつもりで練習して下さい．
■ パニック発作 (panic attack) を訴える患者を想定して会話をしてみましょう．
　下記の用語ファイルを参考にして下さい．

用語ファイル

■パニック発作の一般的な症状

強い不安感にたびたび襲われる	suffer from intense anxiety very often
めまいがする	feel dizzy
吐き気がする	feel nauseous
呼吸が速くなる	breathe rapidly
心臓がドキドキする	have palpitations
震える	tremble
汗が出る	sweat a lot
イライラする	feel irritable

B Medications　　　薬剤投与

■ 患者さんから正確なデータを得るための具体的な表現を集めました．テキストを開いてCDの音声に合わせて発音し，CDのスピードに慣れてきたらテキストを閉じてシャドーイングをしてみましょう．

🎧 44

▶ I'm going to give you some medication for your illness.
治療のための薬をさしあげます．

▶ Let me give you...
1. some tablets.　2. some pills.
3. some powder.　4. a liquid medication.　5. an ointment.
6. a suppository.　7. eyedrops.
8. a medication under your tongue.　9. a compress [poultice].

薬は…でお出しします．
1. 錠剤　2. 丸薬　3. 粉薬　4. 水薬
5. 軟膏　6. 坐薬　7. 点眼薬　8. 舌下錠
9. 湿布薬

— This medication is for ＿＿ days [weeks].
—この薬は…日〔週〕分です．

— You'll take two kinds of medication.
—2種類の飲み薬がでています．

▶ Please take [use] this medication exactly as directed.
薬は指示どおりに飲んで〔使って〕下さい．

▶ This is a prescription for your medication.
これが薬の処方箋です．

— You can have the prescription filled at any outside pharmacy.
—処方箋はどこの院外調剤薬局へ持って行ってもいいですよ．

— Please get your medication from the hospital pharmacy.
—薬は病院内の薬局でもらって下さい．

▶ Please call me [us]...
1. if your symptoms do not improve (within a few days).
2. if your symptoms become worse.

もし…ときは連絡して下さい．
1.（2，3日たっても）症状が改善しない
2. 症状が前よりひどくなる

Lesson 11

3. if you notice any unexpected side effects.
3. 予期しない副作用がみられる

4. if you have any questions.
4. 何かご質問がある

▶ You don't need any medication today.
今日は薬がありません．

▶ That medication is not available in Japan.
（日本では認可されていない薬を要求した場合）その薬は日本では手に入りません．

コラム	頻度の表現
■よく使う表現	
毎時間	every hour
毎日	every day
6 時間ごと	every six hours
4 時間に 1 回	once every four hours
1 日おき	every other day
3 日に 1 回	every three days
1 日〔週〕1 回〔2/3 回〕	once〔twice/three times〕a day〔week〕
朝に	in the morning
食前に	before meals
食後に	after meals
食間に	between meals
就寝時に	at bedtime
必要に応じて	when you need it

Lesson 12 皮膚科

A Skin Rashes (Possible disease: atopic dermatitis)

○● *Let's Listen!* ●○   45

■ 状況を思い浮かべながら，CD を聴きましょう． D/N: Doctor/Nurse   P: Patient

D/N: Good morning. I'm Dr.〔Nurse〕Kaneko. Ms. Kim?
P: That's right.
D/N: Please sit down. Now, how can I help you today?
P: I have a rash on my arms, and it's awfully itchy.
D/N: Where on your arms?
P: Here.
D/N: Anywhere else?
P: I'm having it right here, too.
D/N: How long have you had the rash?
P: It's been about a month or so.
D/N: How did it develop? Suddenly?
P: Oh, no, it developed gradually, and it's been getting worse.
D/N: Does anything make it worse? Exercise or stress?
P: No, I don't think so.
D/N: Have you taken any medications in the past few months?
P: No, I haven't.
D/N: Are you allergic to anything, such as detergent or cosmetics?
P: No, I don't have any allergy to them.
D/N: Have you ever had asthma or hay fever?
P: Yes, I have hay fever every spring.
D/N: Are you taking anything to relieve the itching?
P: I put some over-the-counter cream on the rash, but it doesn't help.
D/N: OK, now I'm going to give you a prescription for a steroid ointment. I want you to apply it once a day after your bath.
P: I understand. Is there anything I should be careful of?
D/N: Avoid scratching your skin. Also, you should take a bath or shower in lukewarm water. And it's important to use a mild soap.

A 湿疹（アトピー性皮膚炎の疑い）

D/N: 医師 / 看護師　　**P:** 患者

- **D/N:** おはようございます．医師〔看護師〕の金子です．キムさんですね．
- **P:** はい，そうです．
- **D/N:** おかけ下さい．どうなさいましたか．
- **P:** 腕に湿疹ができて，すごくかゆいんです．
- **D/N:** 腕のどこですか．
- **P:** ここです．
- **D/N:** ほかの場所には？
- **P:** ここにもあります．
- **D/N:** 湿疹ができてどのくらいになりますか．
- **P:** 1か月くらいです．
- **D/N:** 湿疹の起こり方は...　突然でしたか．
- **P:** いいえ，徐々にできて，ますますひどくなっています．
- **D/N:** 悪化させるものがありますか．運動やストレスなど？
- **P:** いいえ，ないと思います．
- **D/N:** この数か月に服用した薬がありますか．
- **P:** いいえ，飲んでいません．
- **D/N:** アレルギーがありますか．洗剤や化粧品とか？
- **P:** いいえありません．
- **D/N:** 喘息や花粉症にかかったことがありますか．
- **P:** ええ，毎年春に花粉症がでます．
- **D/N:** かゆみを和らげるために何かしていますか．
- **P:** 市販のクリームを使ってみましたが，効き目がありません．
- **D/N:** それではステロイド軟膏を処方しましょう．1日に1回，入浴後に塗って下さい．
- **P:** わかりました．何か気をつけることはありますか．
- **D/N:** 皮膚をかかないようにして下さい．それからお風呂やシャワーはぬるま湯にして下さい．それに低刺激性の石鹸を使うことが重要です．

○● Words and Phrases ●○

- [ ] **skin rash** 皮膚の湿疹
- [ ] **suddenly** 突然
- [ ] **get worse** 悪化する
- [ ] **stress** ストレス
- [ ] **allergy** アレルギー
- [ ] **cosmetics** 化粧品
- [ ] **hay fever** 花粉症
- [ ] **over-the-counter cream** 市販クリーム
- [ ] **steroid ointment** ステロイド軟膏
- [ ] **scratch** ひっかく
- [ ] **lukewarm water** ぬるま湯
- [ ] **itchy** かゆい
- [ ] **gradually** 徐々に
- [ ] **exercise** 運動
- [ ] **allergic** アレルギーのある
- [ ] **detergent** 洗剤
- [ ] **asthma** 喘息
- [ ] **relieve the itching** かゆみを和らげる
- [ ] **prescription** 処方箋
- [ ] **apply** 塗る
- [ ] **bath** 風呂
- [ ] **mild soap** 低刺激性の石鹸

○● Useful Expressions ●○

■ 会話モデルの重要表現を確認しましょう．テキストを開いて CD の音声に合わせて発音し，CD のスピードに慣れてきたらテキストを閉じてシャドーイングしてみましょう．

▶ How long have you had the rash?	湿疹ができてどのくらいになりますか．
▶ How did it develop? Suddenly?	湿疹の起こり方は．．．突然でしたか．
▶ Does anything make it worse? Exercise or stress?	悪化させるものがありますか．運動やストレスなど？
▶ Have you taken any medications in the past few months?	この数か月に服用した薬がありますか．
▶ Are you allergic to anything, such as detergent or cosmetics?	アレルギーがありますか．洗剤や化粧品とか？
▶ Have you ever had asthma or hay fever?	喘息や花粉症にかかったことがありますか．
▶ Are you taking anything to relieve the itching?	かゆみを和らげるために何かしていますか．

▶ OK, now I'm going to give you a prescription for a steroid ointment.

▶ I want you to apply it once a day after your bath.

▶ Avoid scratching your skin.

▶ Also, you should take a bath or shower in lukewarm water.

▶ And it's important to use a mild soap.

それではステロイド軟膏を処方しましょう.

1日に1回, 入浴後に塗って下さい.

皮膚をかかないようにして下さい.

それからお風呂やシャワーはぬるま湯にして下さい.

それに低刺激性の石鹸を使うことが重要です.

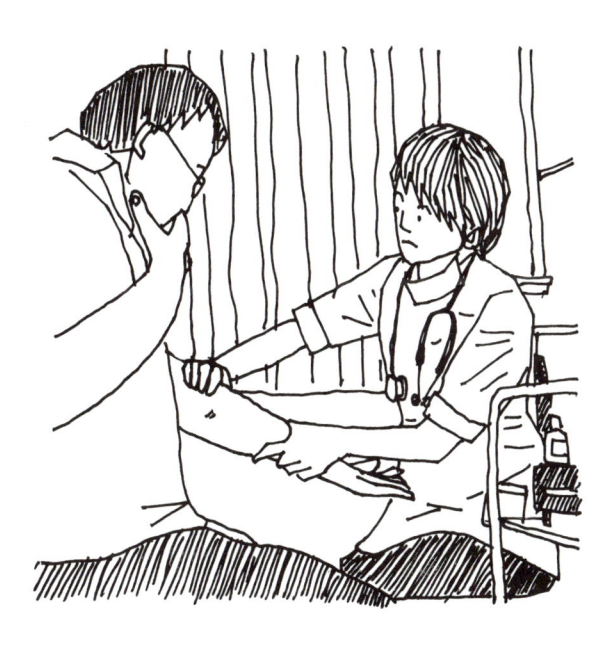

○● **Let's Try!** ●○

■ 会話モデルを参考にして，医師・看護師・患者になったつもりで練習して下さい．
■ 花粉症（hay fever）の症状を訴える患者を想定して会話をしてみましょう．
　下記の用語ファイルを参考にして下さい．

用語ファイル

■花粉症の一般的な症状

鼻水が出る	have a runny nose
鼻がつまる	have a stuffy nose
よくくしゃみが出る	sneeze a lot
目がかゆい	the eyes are itchy
目がゴロゴロする	the eyes feel gritty
涙が出る	have watery eyes
のどが痛む〔かゆい〕	have a sore〔an itchy〕throat
イライラする	feel irritable

B Allergy   アレルギー歴

■ 患者さんから正確なデータを得るための具体的な表現を集めました．テキストを開いてCDの音声に合わせて発音し，CDのスピードに慣れてきたらテキストを閉じてシャドーイングをしてみましょう．

🎧 48

▶ Are you allergic to anything?　　　アレルギーがありますか．

▶ Do you have any allergies?　　　アレルギーがありますか．
— What types of allergies do you have?　　　—どんなアレルギーがありますか．
— Does it occur...　　　—症状は…出ますか．
　1. all the time?　　　1. しょっちゅう
　2. just at certain times of the year?　　　2. ある特定の時期に

▶ Have you ever had asthma〔hay fever〕?　　　これまでに喘息〔花粉症〕になったことがありますか．

▶ What happens to you when you have an allergic reaction?　　　どんなアレルギー反応を起こしますか．
— Do you get...　　　…が起きますか．
　1. a rash?　2. hives?　3. itching?　　　1. 発疹　2. 蕁麻疹　3. かゆみ　4. 腫れ
　4. swelling?　5. a runny nose?　　　5. 鼻水　6. 涙　7. 目のかゆみ　8. 息切れ
　6. watery eyes?　7. itchy eyes?
　8. shortness of breath?

▶ Are you allergic to any medications?　　　薬に対するアレルギーがありますか．
— Which medications?　　　—どの薬に対するアレルギーですか．

▶ Is there anything else you would like to tell me?　　　他にお話になりたいことがありますか．

Lesson 13 産婦人科

A Pregnancy

○● Let's Listen! ●○   49

■ 状況を思い浮かべながら，CD を聴きましょう．　D/M: Doctor/Midwife　P: Patient

D/M: Good morning, Mrs. Shaw. You're now 12 weeks pregnant, aren't you?
P: That's right.
D/M: How have you been since I last saw you? Do you still suffer from morning sickness?
P: No, I'm OK now.
D/M: Does your abdomen feel bloated? Do you have any vaginal bleeding?
P: No, I don't think so.
D/M: OK, now let me examine you and do an ultrasound test.
　　　　………

（診察，超音波検査後に）

D/M: The baby is growing well. The heart is beating strongly.
P: Really? I'm so glad!
D/M: Here's the ultrasound film of your baby. This is for you.
P: Thank you.
D/M: You're welcome. I'd like to ask you about your labor and delivery. Do you want to have the baby in this hospital?
P: Yes, of course.
D/M: Which childbirth method do you prefer? Natural, planned, or painless delivery?
P: Let me see... I prefer a natural delivery.
D/M: Did you get a Boshi-techo, the Mother and Child Health Handbook?
P: No, not yet.
D/M: Then, please go to the health center and get it.
P: OK, I will.
D/M: Your next checkup is February 3rd, Wednesday. Call us if you have any concerns. Please take care of yourself.

A 妊娠

D/M: 医師 / 助産師　P: 患者

D/M: ショーさん，おはようございます．今，妊娠12週ですね．
P: ええ，そうです．
D/M: この前診察してから具合はいかがですか．つわりはまだありますか．

P: いいえ，もう大丈夫です．
D/M: お腹がはっていますか．腟からの出血がありますか．
P: いいえ，ありません．
D/M: それでは診察，それから超音波の検査をしましょう．
　　　………

D/M: 赤ちゃんは順調に大きくなっていますよ．心臓は元気に拍動しています．
P: 本当ですか．うれしい！
D/M: 赤ちゃんの超音波写真です．差し上げます．
P: ありがとうございます．
D/M: どういたしまして．出産についてお尋ねします．この病院での出産を希望されますか．

P: はい，もちろんです．
D/M: どんな方法での出産を希望しますか．自然分娩，計画分娩，無痛分娩など．

P: そうですね...自然分娩で産みたいです．
D/M: 母子手帳はもらいましたか．
P: いいえ，まだです．
D/M: 保健所に行って交付してもらって下さい．
P: はい，そうします．
D/M: 次の検診日は2月3日，水曜日です．心配なことがあったらお電話を下さい．では，お大事に．

○● Words and Phrases ●○

- pregnancy　妊娠
- suffer from　苦しむ
- feel bloated　（お腹が）はる
- labor and delivery　出産［陣痛・分娩］
- prefer　より好む
- planned　計画した
- pregnant　妊娠した
- morning sickness　つわり
- vaginal bleeding　腟からの出血
- childbirth method　出産方法
- natural　自然の
- painless　無痛の

○● Useful Expressions ●○

■ 会話モデルの重要表現を確認しましょう．テキストを開いてCDの音声に合わせて発音し，CDのスピードに慣れてきたらテキストを閉じてシャドーイングしてみましょう．

▶ You're now 12 weeks pregnant, aren't you?	今，妊娠12週ですね．
▶ How have you been since I last saw you?	この前診察してから具合はいかがですか．
▶ Do you still suffer from morning sickness?	つわりはまだありますか．
▶ Does your abdomen feel bloated?	お腹がはっていますか．
▶ Do you have any vaginal bleeding?	腟からの出血がありますか．
▶ The baby is growing well.	赤ちゃんは順調に大きくなっていますよ．
▶ The heart is beating strongly.	心臓は元気に拍動しています．
▶ Here's the ultrasound film of your baby. This is for you.	赤ちゃんの超音波写真です．差し上げます．
▶ I'd like to ask you about your labor and delivery. Do you want to have the baby in this hospital?	出産についてお尋ねします．この病院での出産を希望されますか．

▶ **Which childbirth method do you prefer? Natural, planned, or painless delivery?**

▶ **Your next checkup is February 3rd, Wednesday.**

▶ **Call us if you have any concerns.**

▶ **Please take care of yourself.**

どんな方法での出産を希望しますか．自然分娩，計画分娩，無痛分娩など．

次の検診日は2月3日，水曜日です．

心配なことがあったらお電話を下さい．

では，お大事に．

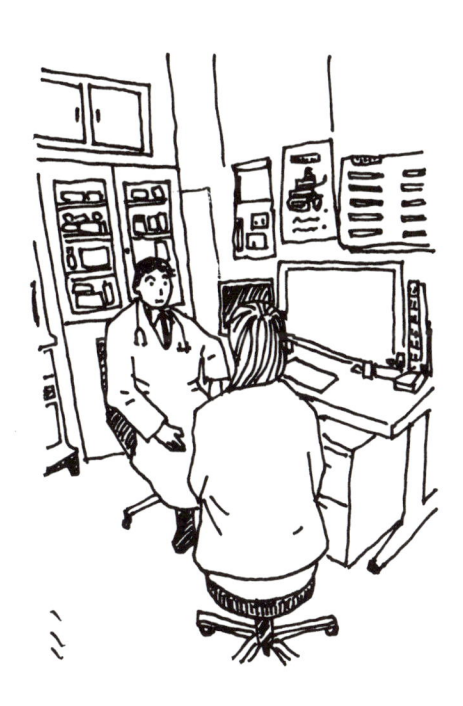

○● *Let's Try!* ●○

■ 会話モデルを参考にして，医師・助産師・患者になったつもりで練習して下さい．
■ 妊娠10週で，つわり（morning sickness）を訴える患者を想定して会話をしてみましょう．
下記の用語ファイルを参考にして下さい．

用語ファイル

■つわりの一般的な症状

体がだるい	feel tired
吐き気がする，特に朝に	feel nauseous, especially in the morning
嘔吐する	vomit［throw up］
食欲がなくなる	lose *one's* appetite
食べ物の好き嫌いが変化する	develop a change in likes and dislikes of certain foods
においに敏感になる	become sensitive to smells

B Obstetric Examination　産科診察

■ 患者さんから正確なデータを得るための具体的な表現を集めました．テキストを開いてCDの音声に合わせて発音し，CDのスピードに慣れてきたらテキストを閉じてシャドーイングをしてみましょう． 🎧52

▶ When was the first day of your last period?　最終月経の初日はいつでしたか．

▶ Do you have〔Have you had〕any...　あなたは…がありますか〔ありましたか〕．
1. nausea?　2. vomiting?　3. loss of appetite?　4. constipation?　5. swelling?
1. 吐き気　2. 嘔吐　3. 食欲不振　4. 便秘　5. むくみ

▶ Have you felt your baby's movement?　赤ちゃんの胎動を感じましたか．

▶ I'm going to〔Let me〕examine you.　診察いたしましょう．

▶ Please lie down on this bed.　このベッドに横になって下さい．

▶ I'm going to〔Let me〕measure your abdominal circumference.　腹囲を測りましょう．

▶ I'm going to〔Let me〕do an ultrasound test.　超音波検査をしましょう．

▶ The baby is supposed to weigh about 1,500 grams.　赤ちゃんの体重は推定1,500グラムです．
— The baby is healthy and well.　—赤ちゃんは元気です．

▶ Would you like to know your baby's sex?　お子さんの性別をお知りになりたいですか．

▶ Please lie down on the exam table.　それでは，診察台にあがって下さい．
— Please remove all your underwear.　—下着はすべて脱いで下さい．
— Open your legs a little for the examination.　—内診をしますので，足を少し開いて下さい．

—**Relax the muscles of your abdomen, and breathe deeply and slowly.**

—お腹の力を抜いてゆっくりと深呼吸して下さい．

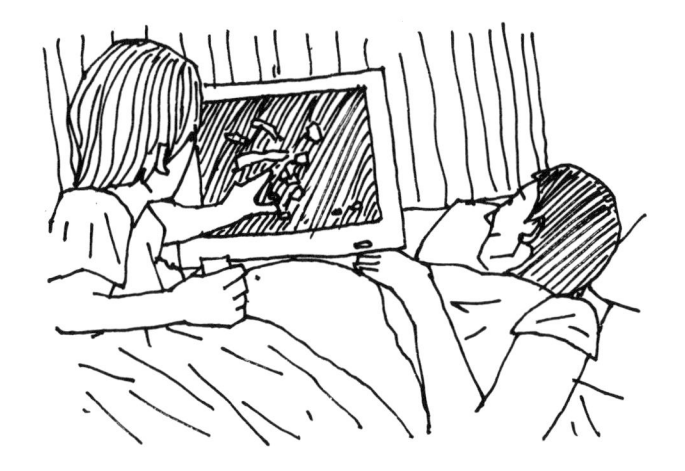

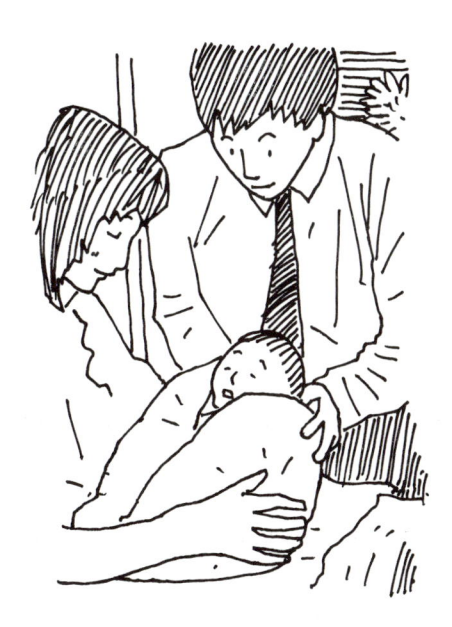

スピーキング攻略のヒント(5)　〜品詞による発音の違い〜

品詞によって綴り字やアクセントの位置が異なることがあるので注意しましょう．
a) 名詞形・動詞形・形容詞形で綴り字や発音が変化します．
　　breath（息）　　　　　⇔ breathe（息をする）
　　blood（血）　　　　　 ⇔ bleed（出血する）
　　nose（鼻）　　　　　　⇔ nasal（鼻の）
b) 名詞形と形容詞形でアクセントの位置が変化します．
　　állergy（アレルギー）　⇔ allérgic（アレルギー性の）
　　ábdomen（腹部）　　　 ⇔ abdóminal（腹部の）
　　álcohol（アルコール）　⇔ alcohólic（アルコール性の）
c) 同じ形ですが，名詞形と動詞形でアクセントの位置が異なります．
　　díscharge（退院・分泌）⇔ dischárge（退院する・分泌する）
　　récord（記録）　　　　 ⇔ recórd（記録する）
　　prógress（進行）　　　 ⇔ progréss（進行する）

Lesson 14　小児科

A Asthma Attacks

○● *Let's Listen!* ●○　　　　　　　　　　　　　53

■ 状況を思い浮かべながら，CD を聴きましょう．**D/N: Doctor/Nurse　M: Mother**

D/N: Hi, Peter. Hello, Mrs. Johnson. How can I help him?
M: He's been wheezy toward dawn for a few days. He coughs a lot and has difficulty breathing.
D/N: Has he had any cold symptoms? Fever or sore throat?
M: No.
D/N: Has he ever been told that he has asthma?
M: Yes, he was first diagnosed as having asthma when he was two years old.
D/N: How often does he have attacks?
M: He had attacks once a month before he started elementary school, but he hasn't had any for a few years.
D/N: Has he been taking any drugs for the asthma?
M: He used to use a steroid inhaler regularly, but in the past few years he hasn't taken anything for asthma.
D/N: Now, let me listen to his chest. Peter, take a deep breath.
　　　………

（診察後に）

D: It seems he's having an asthma attack.
M: Does he have to be hospitalized?
D: I'm not sure yet. First, let's have him inhale a bronchodilator.

A 喘息発作

D/N: 医師 / 看護師　**M:** 患者の母

D/N: こんにちは，ピーター君．こんにちは，ジョンソンさん．どうしましたか．
M: 2，3日前から，明け方にゼイゼイするようになりました．咳が多くて息苦しそうです．

D/N: 風邪の症状はありますか．熱やのどの痛みなど？
M: いいえ，ありません．
D/N: これまでに喘息と言われたことはありますか．
M: 2歳の時に初めて喘息と診断されました．
D/N: 発作の頻度はどのくらいですか．
M: 小学校入学前までは1か月に1度は発作が起きていましたが，この2，3年はほとんど発作がありませんでした．
D/N: 最近，喘息の薬を使用していますか．
M: 以前はステロイドの吸入薬を定期的に使っていましたが，この数年間は何も治療を受けていません．
D/N: それでは，聴診しましょう．ピーター君，深呼吸をして下さい．
　　　　………

D: やはり，喘息の発作のようですね．
M: 入院が必要ですか．
D: まだわかりません．まず気管支拡張薬を吸入してみましょう．

○● Words and Phrases ●○ 🎧54

- [ ] **asthma attack** 喘息発作
- [ ] **dawn** 明け方
- [ ] **elementary school** 小学校
- [ ] **it seems** …のように思われる
- [ ] **bronchodilator** 気管支拡張薬
- [ ] **wheezy** ゼイゼイする
- [ ] **be diagnosed** 診断される
- [ ] **inhaled steroid** ステロイド吸入薬
- [ ] **be hospitalized** 入院する

○● Useful Expressions ●○ 🎧55

■ 会話モデルの重要表現を確認しましょう．テキストを開いてCDの音声に合わせて発音し，CDのスピードに慣れてきたらテキストを閉じてシャドーイングしてみましょう．

▶ Has he had any cold symptoms? Fever or sore throat?	風邪の症状はありますか．熱やのどの痛みなど？
▶ Has he ever been told that he has asthma?	これまでに喘息と言われたことはありますか．
▶ How often does he have attacks?	発作の頻度はどのくらいですか．
▶ Has he been taking any drugs for the asthma?	最近，喘息の薬を使用していますか．
▶ Now, let me listen to his chest.	それでは，聴診しましょう．
▶ Peter, take a deep breath.	ピーター君，深呼吸をして下さい．
▶ It seems he's having an asthma attack.	やはり，喘息の発作のようですね．
▶ I'm not sure yet.	まだわかりません．
▶ First, let's have him inhale a bronchodilator.	まず気管支拡張薬を吸入してみましょう．

○● ***Let's Try!*** ●○

■ 会話モデルを参考にして，医師・看護師・患者の母になったつもりで練習して下さい．
■ 38度の熱と発疹のある幼児を想定して，その母親と会話をしてみましょう．
　下記の用語ファイルを参考にして下さい．

用語ファイル

■水痘（chickenpox）の一般的な症状

軽度の熱がある	have a mild fever
最初，かゆくて，赤い発疹が出る	have itchy, red spots first
体中に水疱ができる	develop small blisters all over the body
かさぶたがある	have scabs

■風疹（rubella）の一般的な症状

軽度の熱がある	have a mild fever
赤またはピンク色のまだらな発疹がある	have a red or pink mottled rash
首のリンパ腺が腫れている	have swollen glands in the neck

B Immunization and Health Checkup   予防接種・健診

■ 患者さんから正確なデータを得るための具体的な表現を集めました．テキストを開いてCDの音声に合わせて発音し，CDのスピードに慣れてきたらテキストを閉じてシャドーイングをしてみましょう． 🎧56

Immunization 予防接種

▶ What vaccinations has he〔she〕had?
これまでにどんな予防接種を受けましたか．

— Let me see the Mother and Child Health Handbook.
—母子（健康）手帳を見せて下さい．

▶ I'm going to give him〔her〕an immunization shot today.
今日は予防注射をしましょう．

— Please hold him〔her〕firmly.
—しっかり抱っこしていて下さい．

— He〔She〕shouldn't exercise hard today.
—今日は激しい運動は控えて下さい．

— He〔She〕can have a bath.
—お風呂に入ってもいいですよ．

— He〔She〕may have some slight swelling, but don't worry.
—少し腫れるかもしれませんが，心配ないでしょう．

— Please call us if you have any concerns.
—心配なときはお電話下さい．

▶ The next vaccination will be one month from now.
次回の予防接種は1か月後です．

Health Checkup 健診

▶ When was his〔her〕last health checkup?
前回の健診はいつでしたか．

— Have you been told that he〔she〕has a problem?
—何か異常所見はありましたか．

— What was the problem?
—何の異常ですか．

— **What kind of instructions or treatments did he〔she〕get?** 　—どのような指導，治療を受けましたか．

▶ **Has he〔she〕had an exam by a specialist?** 　専門医の診察を受けたことがありますか．
— **When was it?** 　—いつですか．
— **What did the doctor tell you about his〔her〕problem?** 　—何と言われましたか．

▶ **His〔Her〕4-month〔18-month/3-year〕health checkup is Tuesday, June 7th.** 　4か月〔18か月/3年〕健診は6月7日，火曜日です．
— **Please check the schedule in your city bulletin.** 　—市の広報で予定をチェックして下さい．

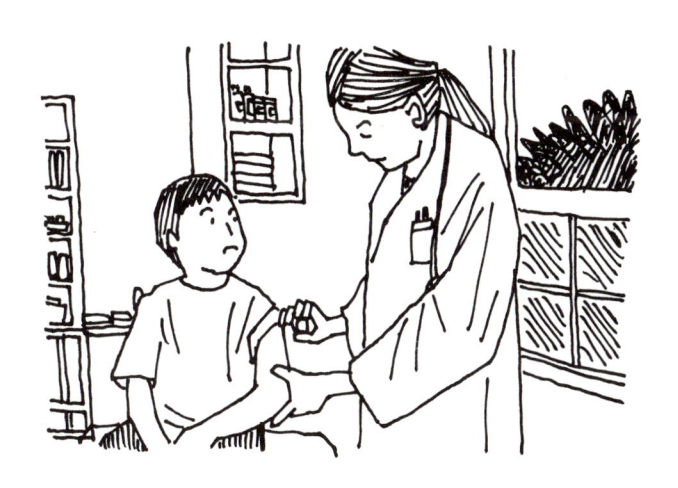

Lesson 15　会計窓口

A Bill Payment

○● *Let's Listen!* ●○　　　57

■ 状況を思い浮かべながら，CD を聴きましょう． **C: Cashier**　**P: Patient**

C： Mr. Tom Katz, please come to Window 6.
　………

C: Are you Mr. Tom Katz?
P: Yes, that's right.
C: You don't have insurance, so you'll have to pay all your medical expenses.
P: Is that so? But I have travel insurance.
C: I'm afraid we can't accept your travel insurance.
P: I see. How much do I have to pay?
C: Let me see... Your bill is 21,000 yen.
P: OK. I have to submit an itemized statement and receipt to the travel insurance company for reimbursement. Could you give me an itemized bill?
C: Yes, of course. Would you like to pay your bill in full or make a 5,000 yen deposit now and pay the difference later?
P: I'll pay it in full now. Do you accept credit cards?
C: Sure. Wait a minute, please. ... Here are your itemized bill and receipt.

P: Thank you. And could I have a copy of my medical records?
C: Yes, medical records are available upon request. But it will take a few weeks. We will either mail them to you or you may pick them up at our office.

A 診療費の支払い

C: 会計係　P: 患者

C:　トム・キャッツさん，6番窓口においで下さい．
　　………

C:　トム・キャッツさんですね．
P:　はい，そうです．
C:　保険をお持ちでないので自費診療になります．
P:　えっ，そうですか．旅行保険があるのですが．
C:　残念ですが，あなたの旅行保険は扱えないんですよ．
P:　わかりました．おいくらになりますか．
C:　えーと，請求額は 21,000 円になります．
P:　わかりました．旅行保険会社に払い戻しのため明細書と領収書を提出しなければならないので，明細書のついた請求書をいただけませんか．

C:　はい，お出しします．全額お支払いになりますか．あるいは，5,000 円の保証金をおいて，差額はあとでお支払いになりますか．
P:　今，全額払います．クレジットカードでいいですか．
C:　もちろん，けっこうです．ちょっとお待ち下さい．... 明細書つきの請求書と領収書です．
P:　ありがとう．それに，診療記録のコピーがほしいのですが．
C:　はい，診療記録はご要望によりお出しします．ただ 2，3 週間かかります．郵送でも，こちらに取りに来て下さってもけっこうです．

○● Words and Phrases ●○ 　　　　　　　　　　　　　　　　　🎧58

- [ ] **insurance** 保険
- [ ] **travel insurance** 旅行保険
- [ ] **bill** 請求書
- [ ] **reimbursement** 払い戻し
- [ ] **in full** 全額で
- [ ] **credit card** クレジットカード
- [ ] **medical record** 診療記録
- [ ] **upon request** 要望があれば
- [ ] **medical expenses** 医療費
- [ ] **I'm afraid** 残念ですが...
- [ ] **receipt** 領収書
- [ ] **deposit** 保証金
- [ ] **difference** 差(額)
- [ ] **itemized bill** 明細書つきの請求書
- [ ] **available** 入手できる

○● Useful Expressions ●○ 　　　　　　　　　　　　　　　　🎧59

■ 会話モデルの重要表現を確認しましょう．テキストを開いてCDの音声に合わせて発音し，CDのスピードに慣れてきたらテキストを閉じてシャドーイングしてみましょう．

▶ You don't have insurance, so you'll have to pay all your medical expenses.	保険をお持ちでないので自費診療になります．
▶ I'm afraid we can't accept your travel insurance.	残念ですが，あなたの旅行保険は扱えないんですよ．
▶ Let me see... Your bill is 21,000 yen.	えーと，請求額は21,000円になります．
▶ Yes, of course. Would you like to pay your bill in full or make a 5,000 yen deposit now and pay the difference later?	はい，お出しします．全額お支払いになりますか．あるいは，5,000円の保証金をおいて，差額はあとでお支払いになりますか．
▶ Sure. Wait a minute, please. ... Here are your itemized bill and receipt.	もちろん，けっこうです．ちょっとお待ち下さい．...　明細書つきの請求書と領収書です．
▶ Yes, medical records are available upon request. But it will take a few weeks.	はい，診療記録はご要望によりお出しします．ただ2, 3週間かかります．

▶ We will either mail them to you or you may pick them up at our office.

郵送でも，こちらに取りに来て下さってもけっこうです．

○● Let's Try! ●○

■ 会話モデルを参考にして，会計係・患者になったつもりで練習して下さい．
■ 医療費支払いの会話に続けて，薬の受け取り方を患者に説明してみましょう．
　下記の用語ファイルを参考にして下さい．

用語ファイル

■処方箋(prescription)について

薬は薬局でもらう	pick up the medication at a pharmacy
処方箋を薬局の窓口に出す	give the prescription at the pharmacy counter
院外の調剤薬局で処方薬を調合してもらう	have the prescription filled at an outside pharmacy
院内の薬局でもらう	get the medication from the hospital pharmacy

B Health Insurance and Payment　保険・支払い

■ 患者さんから正確なデータを得るための具体的な表現を集めました．テキストを開いてCDの音声に合わせて発音し，CDのスピードに慣れてきたらテキストを閉じてシャドーイングをしてみましょう．

🎧 60

Health Insurance　保険

▶ Let me ask you about your insurance.　保険についておうかがいします．

▶ Do you have Japanese health insurance〔overseas travel insurance/other public〔private〕assistance〕?　日本の健康保険〔海外旅行保険/他の公的〔私的〕援助〕がありますか．

▶ Do you have an insurance card?　保険証をもっていますか．
— Please show it to me.　—それを見せて下さい．
— Please be sure to bring it next time you come.　—次回に必ず持参して下さい．

▶ If you don't have insurance, you'll have to pay all your medical expenses.　保険がないと自費診療になります．

▶ I'm sorry, but we can't accept foreign insurance at our hospital.　申し訳ありませんが，当院では外国の保険は扱えません．

Payment　支払い

▶ How will you pay the hospital fees?　病院の費用は何でお支払いになりますか．
— Cash〔Credit card〕?　—現金〔カード〕ですか．
— Please bring your company's insurance claim form next time you come.　—次回のとき保険金支払い申請書をもってきて下さい．

| コラム | 医学専門用語と一般語 |

外国人患者さんを前にして医療スタッフは，その患者さんがどの程度の医学知識を持っているかを測りかねて戸惑うかもしれません．例えば，

[専門用語]
myocardial infarction（心筋梗塞）
cerebrovascular accident（脳血管障害）
dyspepsia（消化不良）
hemorrhage（出血）
myopia（近視）
tinnitus（耳鳴り）
hypertension（高血圧）
hypotension（低血圧）

[一般語]
heart attack（心臓発作）
stroke（脳卒中）
indigestion
bleeding
nearsightedness
ringing in the ears
high blood pressure
low blood pressure

患者さんによっては heart attack という一般語よりも，myocardial infarction のほうが正確でわかりやすいかもしれませんが，英語を話す外国人患者がすべて英語を母語としているとは限りません．たとえ英語が母語の人にとっても，医学用語は特殊で理解するのは困難です．患者さんと話すときにはできるだけ平易な一般語を使うようにしたいものです．

Lesson 16　病院のなかの基礎用語

1　診療部門

■ 診療部門

- ☐ general medicine　　　　　　　　　　☐ 総合診療科
- ☐ internal medicine　　　　　　　　　　☐ 内科
  - ☐ general internal medicine　　　　　☐ 一般内科
  - ☐ respiratory medicine　　　　　　　☐ 呼吸器内科
  - ☐ cardiology　　　　　　　　　　　　☐ 循環器内科
  - ☐ gastroenterology　　　　　　　　　☐ 消化器内科
  - ☐ metabolism and endocrinology　　　☐ 代謝・内分泌内科
  - ☐ nephrology　　　　　　　　　　　　☐ 腎臓内科
  - ☐ neurology[neurosciences]　　　　　☐ 神経内科
  - ☐ hematology　　　　　　　　　　　　☐ 血液内科
  - ☐ rheumatology and clinical immunology　☐ リウマチ・膠原病内科
  - ☐ geriatrics　　　　　　　　　　　　☐ 老年内科
  - ☐ psychosomatic medicine　　　　　　☐ 心療内科
- ☐ surgery　　　　　　　　　　　　　　☐ 外科
  - ☐ general surgery　　　　　　　　　　☐ 一般外科
  - ☐ cardiovascular surgery　　　　　　☐ 心臓血管外科
  - ☐ thoracic surgery　　　　　　　　　☐ 呼吸器外科
  - ☐ gastroenterological surgery　　　　☐ 消化器外科
  - ☐ breast and endocrine surgery　　　☐ 乳腺・内分泌外科
  - ☐ neurosurgery　　　　　　　　　　　☐ 脳神経外科
  - ☐ orthopedic surgery　　　　　　　　☐ 整形外科
  - ☐ plastic surgery　　　　　　　　　　☐ 形成外科
  - ☐ pediatric surgery　　　　　　　　　☐ 小児外科
- ☐ pediatrics　　　　　　　　　　　　　☐ 小児科
- ☐ obstetrics　　　　　　　　　　　　　☐ 産科

- ☐ **gynecology** ☐ 婦人科
- ☐ **urology** ☐ 泌尿器科
- ☐ **psychiatry** ☐ 精神科
- ☐ **ophthalmology** ☐ 眼科
- ☐ **otorhinolaryngology** ☐ 耳鼻咽喉科
   ENT（ear, nose, and throat）
- ☐ **dermatology** ☐ 皮膚科
- ☐ **radiology** ☐ 放射線科
- ☐ **anesthesiology** ☐ 麻酔科
- ☐ **diagnostic pathology** ☐ 病理診断科
- ☐ **dentistry** ☐ 歯科
- ☐ **oral（and maxillofacial）surgery** ☐ 口腔外科
- ☐ **emergency and critical care** ☐ 救急部
- ☐ **rehabilitation** ☐ リハビリテーション科
- ☐ **comprehensive physical examination center, health screening center** ☐ 人間ドック・健診センター

2 病院関係者

■ 1. 専門職

- [ ] physician　　　　　　　　　　　　　　[ ] 医師
  - [ ] internist[physician]　　　　　　　[ ] 内科医
  - [ ] surgeon　　　　　　　　　　　　　　[ ] 外科医
  - [ ] resident　　　　　　　　　　　　　[ ] 研修医
  - [ ] doctor in charge　　　　　　　　　[ ] 担当医
- [ ] dentist　　　　　　　　　　　　　　　[ ] 歯科医
- [ ] nurse　　　　　　　　　　　　　　　　[ ] 看護師
- [ ] pharmacist　　　　　　　　　　　　　[ ] 薬剤師
- [ ] dietician[nutritionist]　　　　　　　[ ] 栄養士
- [ ] medical[clinical]social worker　　　[ ] 医療ソーシャルワーカー
- [ ] psychiatric social worker　　　　　　[ ] 精神保健福祉士
- [ ] radiologic technologist[technician]　[ ] 放射線技師
- [ ] medical technologist[MT]　　　　　　[ ] 臨床検査技師
- [ ] medical engineer　　　　　　　　　　[ ] 臨床工学技士
- [ ] rehabilitation therapist　　　　　　[ ] 療法士
  - [ ] occupational therapist[OT]　　　　[ ] 作業療法士
  - [ ] physical therapist[PT]　　　　　　[ ] 理学療法士
  - [ ] speech-language-hearing therapist[ST]　[ ] 言語聴覚士
- [ ] paramedic[emergency medical technician]　[ ] 救急救命士

■ 2. サービス職

- [ ] hospital attendant, (男性の) orderly　[ ] 介護員
- [ ] nursing assistant[nurse's aide]　　　[ ] 看護助手
- [ ] guard　　　　　　　　　　　　　　　　[ ] 警備員
- [ ] cleaner[cleaning man〔woman〕]　　　　[ ] 清掃員
- [ ] janitor　　　　　　　　　　　　　　　[ ] 用務員

■ 3. 事務職

- ☐ (general office) clerk　　　　☐ 一般事務（職員）
- ☐ receptionist　　　　　　　　☐ 受付事務（職員）
- ☐ unit clerk　　　　　　　　　☐ 病棟事務（職員）
- ☐ cashier　　　　　　　　　　☐ 会計係

■ 4. 管理職

- ☐ president [hospital administrator]　☐ 院長
- ☐ vice president　　　　　　　☐ 副院長
- ☐ medical director for physicians　☐ 診療部長
- ☐ the head (of the ＿＿ Department)　☐ 科長（…科の）
- ☐ director of nursing　　　　　☐ 看護部長
- ☐ head nurse　　　　　　　　☐ 看護主任［主任看護師］
- ☐ director of pharmacy　　　　☐ 薬剤部長
- ☐ director of the administration department　☐ 事務長

■ 5. その他

- ☐ nursing student　　　　　　☐ 看護学生
- ☐ medical student　　　　　　☐ 医学生
- ☐ volunteer　　　　　　　　　☐ ボランティア
- ☐ chaplain　　　　　　　　　☐ （病院付きの）牧師

3 病名

■ 1. 循環器科

- [ ] **high blood pressure**　　　　　　　　　　　[ ] 高血圧
- [ ] **irregular pulse[arrhythmia]**　　　　　　[ ] 不整脈
- [ ] **angina pectoris**　　　　　　　　　　　　[ ] 狭心症
- [ ] **heart attack[myocardial infarction]**　　[ ] 心臓発作[心筋梗塞]
- [ ] **heart failure**　　　　　　　　　　　　　[ ] 心不全
- [ ] **varicose veins** *　　　　　　　　　　　　[ ] 静脈瘤

■ 2. 呼吸器科

- [ ] **common cold syndrome**　　　　　　　　　[ ] かぜ症候群
- [ ] **bronchitis**　　　　　　　　　　　　　　[ ] 気管支炎
- [ ] **pneumonia**　　　　　　　　　　　　　　[ ] 肺炎
- [ ] **influenza**　　　　　　　　　　　　　　 [ ] インフルエンザ
- [ ] **whooping cough[pertussis]**　　　　　　 [ ] 百日咳
- [ ] **pulmonary tuberculosis**　　　　　　　　[ ] 肺結核
- [ ] **asthma**　　　　　　　　　　　　　　　 [ ] 気管支喘息
- [ ] **hyperventilation syndrome**　　　　　　 [ ] 過換気症候群
- [ ] **sleep apnea syndrome**　　　　　　　　　[ ] 睡眠時無呼吸症候群

■ 3. 消化器科

- [ ] **gastritis**　　　　　　　　　　　　　　 [ ] 胃炎
- [ ] **stomach ulcer[gastric ulcer]**　　　　　[ ] 胃潰瘍
- [ ] **appendicitis**　　　　　　　　　　　　　[ ] 虫垂炎
- [ ] **peritonitis**　　　　　　　　　　　　　 [ ] 腹膜炎
- [ ] **piles[hemorrhoids** *]　　　　　　　　　[ ] 痔核
- [ ] **constipation**　　　　　　　　　　　　　[ ] 便秘
- [ ] **fatty liver**　　　　　　　　　　　　　 [ ] 脂肪肝
- [ ] **gallstone**　　　　　　　　　　　　　　 [ ] 胆石

*通例，複数形で用いる．

- [ ] hepatitis   [ ] 肝炎
  — hepatitis B   — B 型肝炎
  — hepatitis C   — C 型肝炎

4. 代謝・内分泌科

- [ ] diabetes (mellitus)   [ ] 糖尿病
- [ ] dyslipidemia   [ ] 脂質異常症
- [ ] gout   [ ] 痛風
- [ ] hypothyroidism   [ ] 甲状腺機能低下症
- [ ] mastopathy   [ ] 乳腺症

5. 血液科

- [ ] iron-deficiency anemia   [ ] 鉄欠乏性貧血
- [ ] leukemia   [ ] 白血病

6. 神経科

- [ ] stroke   [ ] 脳卒中
- [ ] meningitis   [ ] 髄膜炎
- [ ] encephalitis   [ ] 脳炎

7. 精神科

- [ ] Alzheimer-type dementia   [ ] アルツハイマー型認知症
- [ ] insomnia   [ ] 不眠症
- [ ] depression   [ ] うつ病
- [ ] neurosis   [ ] 神経症
- [ ] epilepsy   [ ] てんかん
- [ ] mental retardation   [ ] 精神遅滞

8. 整形外科

- ☐ rheumatoid arthritis ☐ 関節リウマチ
- ☐ intervertebral disk hernia ☐ 椎間板ヘルニア
- ☐ whiplash injury ☐ むち打ち症
- ☐ osteoporosis ☐ 骨粗鬆症
- ☐ dislocation ☐ 脱臼
- ☐ fracture ☐ 骨折

9. 皮膚科

- ☐ prickly heat ☐ あせも[汗疹]
- ☐ eczema ☐ 湿疹
- ☐ acne ☐ にきび[痤瘡]
- ☐ atopic dermatitis ☐ アトピー性皮膚炎
- ☐ baldness[alopecia] ☐ 脱毛症
- ☐ shingles[herpes zoster] ☐ 帯状疱疹
- ☐ drug eruption[drug rash] ☐ 薬疹
- ☐ athlete's foot[tinea pedis] ☐ 水虫[足白癬]

10. 泌尿器科

- ☐ cystitis ☐ 膀胱炎
- ☐ urinary stone ☐ 尿路結石
- ☐ kidney stone ☐ 腎結石
- ☐ enlargement of prostate gland [prostatic hypertrophy] ☐ 前立腺肥大
- ☐ STD[sexually transmitted disease] ☐ 性行為感染症

11. 産婦人科

- ☐ infertility ☐ 不妊症

Lesson 16

- ☐ morning sickness[nausea and vomiting in pregnancy]　☐ つわり[妊娠悪阻]
- ☐ abnormal genital bleeding　☐ 不正性器出血
- ☐ endometritis　☐ 子宮内膜炎
- ☐ uterus myoma　☐ 子宮筋腫

■ 12. 耳鼻咽喉科

- ☐ hay fever　☐ 花粉症
- ☐ allergic rhinitis　☐ アレルギー性鼻炎
- ☐ sinusitis　☐ 副鼻腔炎
- ☐ middle-ear infection[otitis media]　☐ 中耳炎
- ☐ Ménière's disease　☐ メニエール病
- ☐ sudden hearing loss　☐ 突発性難聴
- ☐ enlarged tonsils*　☐ 扁桃肥大

■ 13. 眼科

- ☐ conjunctivitis　☐ 結膜炎
- ☐ nearsightedness[myopia]　☐ 近視
- ☐ farsightedness[hyperopia]　☐ 遠視
- ☐ distorted vision[astigmatism]　☐ 乱視
- ☐ eyestrain　☐ 眼精疲労
- ☐ floaters[muscae volitantes]*　☐ 飛蚊症
- ☐ cataract　☐ 白内障
- ☐ glaucoma　☐ 緑内障

■ 14. 歯科

- ☐ tooth decay[dental caries*]　☐ う歯
- ☐ periodontal disease　☐ 歯周病

15. 小児科

- roseola [exanthema subitum]　□ 突発性発疹
- measles　□ 麻疹
- chickenpox　□ 水痘
- rubella　□ 風疹
- mumps　□ 流行性耳下腺炎
- inguinal hernia　□ 鼠径ヘルニア

索引

欧文

B 型肝炎　105
C 型肝炎　105
CT　41, **45**, 61
E メールアドレス　7
ID バンド　66
MRI　**45**, 61
X 線　41, **44**, 49

あ

あいさつ　**9**
青白い, 顔が　37
仰向け　19, 27
赤い　23
赤さび色　23
赤ちゃん　81, 85
赤みがかった　30, 49
アキレス腱　43
明け方　89
朝　73
足　43
脚　43
足がつる　43
足首　43
足の指　43
汗が出る　71
あせも［汗疹］　106
頭　41
頭が痛い　21
悪化　13, 75
扱う　95
圧迫　45
圧迫感　19
アトピー性皮膚炎　75, 106
歩きにくい　61
アルコール　28, 27
アルコール消毒　39

アルツハイマー型認知症
　　　　　　　　　　105
アレルギー　75, **79**, 87
アレルギー性鼻炎　107
アレルギー反応　39, 45, 79
泡状の　23

い

胃　27, 44
「イー」と言って　24
胃炎　104
胃潰瘍　27, 104
医学生　103
息　24, 87
　──を吸う　24, 31, 44, 46,
　　52
　──を止める　44, 46, 52
　──を吐く　24
息切れ　9, 21, 37, 79
息苦しい　21, 89
胃薬　27
医師　102
意識　41
異常　92
痛み　15, **17**, 49, 55
　──, のどの　89
　──, 胸の　15
　──, 焼き付くような　51
　──の起こり方　17
　──のスケール　17
　──の程度　17
　──の頻度　17
　──のレベル　17
胃痛　28, 33
一過性　13
一般外科　100
一般事務（職員）　103
一般内科　100
いつも　17
遺伝　35

犬が吠えるような　23
胃もたれ　69
イライラ　71, 78
医療ソーシャルワーカー
　　　　　　　　　　102
医療費　96
入れ歯　46
色, 痰の　23
色, 便の　30
違和感　19
院長　103
インフルエンザ　104

う

受付　**3**
受付事務（職員）　103
う歯　107
疑い　55
うつ病　105
腕　43
膿　23
運動　15, 75, 92

え

栄養士　102
エコー　52
遠視　107
援助　98
鉛筆状の　30

お

嘔吐　64, 84, 85
押される　52
お座り下さい　9
お大事に　81
お腹　31
おなら　32
お待たせしました　9

親指　39

か

カード　98
海外旅行保険　98
会計係　103
介護員　102
外国の保険　98
改善しない　72
かかと　43
かかりつけ医　3
過換気症候群　104
かく, 皮膚を　75
確認する　11
確率　35
かさぶた　91
風邪　21, 89
かぜ症候群　104
家族　15, 55
肩　15
硬い　30
固まっている　30
科長（…科の）　103
活字体　3
下半身　32
カフ　18
花粉症　75, **78**, 79
我慢　32
我慢できるほどの　17
かゆい　91
かゆみ　75
かゆみ, 目の　78, 79
空咳　23
体中　91
体の調子　15
軽い　17, 23
渇く　35
肝炎　105
眼科　101
間欠性の　17
看護学生　103
看護師　102
看護主任　103
看護助手　102
看護部長　103
眼精疲労　107

関節リウマチ　106
冠動脈バイパス術　59
丸薬　72
緩和　13

き

黄色味　23
既往　49
気管支炎　104
気管支拡張薬　89
気管支喘息（喘息も参照）
　　　　　　　　　　104
聞き取れない　3
効き目　75
効く　9
聞こえない　64
規則的　69
貴重品　65
気づく　12
記入する　3
気分が悪い　3
希望する　81
救急救命士　102
救急部　101
急性胃炎　27
急性気管支炎　21
急性の　17
吸入　89
吸入薬　89
狭心症　15, 104
胸痛　**15**
胸背部　24
胸部　44, 45
記録　87
緊急連絡先　7, 65
近視　99, 107
金属製品　46
勤務先　7

く

具合　9, 12, 81
具合が悪い　9
空腹の　28
駆血帯　38
くしゃみ　78

薬　9, 27, 65, **72**, 73, 75, 79, 97
管　32, 38
靴下　19
首　44
クリーム, 市販の　75
繰り返し　17
クリップ　45
ぐるぐる回る　64
クレジットカード　95
黒い　30
詳しく話す　15

け

軽快傾向　13
計画分娩　81
形成外科　100
頸椎　44
軽度　91
警備員　102
外科　100
外科医　102
下剤　45
化粧品　75
血圧　15, **18**
血液検査　35, **38**, 49
血液内科　100
月経　**58**
　—— 期間　58
　—— 周期　58
　—— 痛　58
血糖値　35
血尿　49
ゲップ　32, 44
結膜炎　107
下痢　27
原因　13
元気　15
現金　98
健康保険　98
言語聴覚士　102
検査着　32
検査結果　55
検査台　19, 45
検査部位　46
研修医　102
健診　**35**, 49, 92, 93

健診センター　101
検診日　81
検尿　38

こ

口腔外科　101
高血圧　99, 104
甲状腺　52
甲状腺機能低下症　105
香辛料　27
広報, 市の　93
呼吸　71
呼吸器外科　100
呼吸器内科　100
国籍　6
腰　43
個人に関する一般情報　**6**
骨折　43, 106
骨粗鬆症　106
コップ　38, 44
粉薬　72
こぶ　41
コンコンする　23

さ

採血　38
最終月経　55, 58, 85
サイン　59
差額　95
坂道　15
作業療法士　102
酒　27
差し込む　49
坐薬　72
さらさらした　23
産科　100
産科診察　**85**
残尿感　51
残念　95

し

歯科　101
歯科医　102
次回　92, 98

痔核　104
時間帯　12
子宮筋腫　107
子宮内膜炎　107
しこり　31, **55**
持参　98
指示どおり　72
歯周病　107
自然分娩　81
持続時間, 期間　13
持続性　13, 17
下着　18, 85
自宅　7
しっかり　92
湿疹　75, 106
じっと立つ　61
湿布薬　72
質問　6, 59
指導　93
しばしば　17
支払い　**98**
支払う　95
耳鼻咽喉科　101
自費診療　95, 98
しびれる　61
脂質異常症　105
脂肪肝　104
事務長　103
締めつけられる　15
シャワー　75
周期性の　17
住所　7
就寝時　73
手術　**59**
受診　41
出血　61, 81, 87, 99
出血量　58
出産　81
出生地　6
出身　6
種類　12
循環器内科　100
瞬時の　17
順調　81
紹介　**3**, 55
紹介状　3
消化管　32

消化器外科　100
消化器内科　100
小学校　89
消化不良　99
錠剤　72
症状　**12**, 21, 27, 35, 41, 61,
　　　69, 72, 79, 89
　──の起こり方　13
　──の緩和因子　13
　──の経過　13
　──の経験, 同様の　13
　──の増悪因子　13
　──の特徴　12
　──の部位　12
　──の誘発因子　13
少々の　23
小児科　100
小児外科　100
上半身　32
上部消化管内視鏡　32
静脈瘤　104
食後　73
触診　27, 31, 55
食前　73
職場　69
食欲　9, 35, 69, 84
食欲不振　85
初経年齢　58
徐々に　13, 75
初診　3
食間　73
初日　85
処方　27, 75
処方箋　72, **97**
処方薬　97
白い　30
白っぽい　23
心筋梗塞　99, 104
神経症　105
神経内科　100
腎結石　49, 106
進行　87
人工関節　45
深呼吸　86, 89
診察　3, **24**, 31
診察室　3, **9**
診察台　31, 85

申請書　98
親戚　35
心臓　15, 24, 45, 52, 71, 81
心臓血管外科　100
腎臓内科　100
心臓発作　15, 99
診断される　89
心電図　15, **18**
心配　41, 92
心不全　104
蕁麻疹　79
診療記録　95
心療内科　100
診療費　95
診療部長　103

す

推定　85
水痘　**91**, 108
随伴症状　13
水分　45
水疱　91
髄膜炎　105
睡眠　69
睡眠時無呼吸症候群　104
好き嫌い　84
頭痛　21
酸っぱい臭い　30
ステロイド　89
ステロイド軟膏　75
ストッキング　19
ストレス　75

せ

姓　3
正確　49, 55
請求額　95
請求書　95
整形外科　100
生検　32
性行為感染症　106
精神科　101
精神遅滞　105
精神保健福祉士　102
ゼイゼイする　23, 89

清掃員　102
生年月日　6
性別　85
精密検査　55
咳　**21, 23,** 89
　——の種類　23
　——の程度　23
舌下錠　72
石鹸　75
摂氏　18
説明　65
背中　24, 49
　——を押す　24
　——を叩く　24
前回　92
全額　95
洗剤　75
喘息　75, 79, 104
喘息発作　**89**
専門医　55, 93
前立腺肥大　106

そ

造影剤　45, 46
総合診療科　100
装飾品　44, 46
鼠径ヘルニア　108

た

タール様　30
退院　87
体温　18
滞在　7
代謝・内分泌内科　100
体重　35, **69,** 85
大丈夫　32
帯状疱疹　106
大腿　43
大腸内視鏡　32
たいてい　17
胎動　85
耐えられないほどの　17
多少　52
立ちくらみ　37
脱臼　43, 106

抱っこ　92
脱毛症　106
打撲傷　43
だるい　37, 69, 84
痰　21, **23**
　——の色　23
　——の種類　23
胆石　104
担当医　66, 102
担当看護師　66

ち

血　87
血がにじむ　23
血のつながった家族　55
力が入らない　61
力を抜く　38, 86
チクチク　61
乳首　55
腟　81
茶色　30
中耳炎　107
注射　32
虫垂炎　104
虫垂切除術　59
中程度の　17, 23
超音波　49, **52,** 81, 85
徴候　13
調剤薬局, 院外の　97
聴診　**24,** 89
　——, 心臓の　15
　——, 胸の　21
治療　13, 93

つ

椎間板ヘルニア　106
痛風　49, 105
通訳　5, 65
疲れる　35, 37
付き添い　65
突き指　43
つづる　6
つわり　81

て

手　43
手当て　41
手洗い　35
定期的　55, 89
低血圧　99
低刺激性　75
泥状の　30
程度　12
テープ　11
適応障害　69
手首　43, 66
鉄欠乏性貧血　105
徹夜　69
手の指　43
てんかん　105
点眼薬　72
転倒　41
電話番号　7

と

同意　59
同意書　59
どういたしまして　27
動悸　37
どうなさいましたか　9, 21
糖尿病　35, 105
頭部　45, 61
頭部外傷　**41**
透明　23
時々　17
ドキドキする　71
特定の時期　79
時計　46
年　6
突然　13, 51, 75
突然の　17
突発性難聴　107
突発性発疹　108
取りに来る　95
トレッドミル　19
どろどろした　23
鈍痛　28

な

内科　100
内科医　102
内視鏡検査　**32**
内診　85
名前　6
涙　78, 79
軟膏　72

に

におい　84
にきび[痤瘡]　106
肉離れ　43
濁る　49, 51
二重に見える　61
日本　7
日本語　5
入院　59, 61, **65**, 66, 89
入院受付係　65, 66
入院説明書　65
乳癌　55
乳腺症　105
乳腺・内分泌外科　100
乳房　52, 55
乳房温存術　59
乳房自己触診　55
入浴　55, 75
尿　35, 38, 49, 51
尿意　51
尿検査　**38**, 49
尿酸値　49
尿路結石　106
人間ドック　101
妊娠　**81**

ぬ

脱ぐ　18, 85
塗る　75
ぬるま湯　75

ね

熱　**18**, 21, 69, 89, 91
寝つき　69
ねばねばした　23
寝間着　66
眠れない　21
捻挫　43
念のために　32
年齢　6

の

脳炎　105
脳血管障害　99
脳出血　61
脳神経外科　100
脳卒中　99, 105
のど　21, 35, 78
飲み薬　72

は

肺　24
灰色　23
肺炎　104
肺結核　104
バイタルサイン　**18**
配置換え　69
排尿　49
排尿時　51
背部痛　49
測る　18, 85
吐き気　27, 49, 69, 85
拍動　81
白内障　107
白内障手術　59
激しい　15, 17, 23, 49
初めて　61
場所　12
発音　11
発音する　3
白血病　105
発症時刻, 時期　12
鼻　87
鼻がつまる　21, 78
鼻水　78, 79
パニック発作　**71**
払い戻し　95
腹ばい　52

バランス　61
バリウム　44
はる,お腹が　81
腫れ　79
腫れる　91,92
判断　41
バンドエイド　39

ひ

控える　92
膝　43
肘　43
左向き　31,52
ひっかく　76
ひっこめる,お腹を　52
必要に応じて　73
ひどい　23,72
泌尿器科　101
皮膚　39
皮膚科　101
飛蚊症　107
冷や汗　49
百日咳　104
費用,病院の　98
病室　66
病棟　66
病棟事務(職員)　103
病理診断科　101
病歴　12
疲労　69
敏感　84
ピンク色　23
貧血　37
頻度　13,**73**
頻繁に　17

ふ

不安感　71
風疹　**91**,108
腹囲　85
副院長　103
副作用　73
腹痛　**27**,33,69
副鼻腔炎　107
腹部　28,**31**,44,45,52,87

腹膜炎　104
服用　27
ふくらはぎ　43
ふくらませる,お腹を　52
服を着る　32
服を脱ぐ　32
婦人科　101
不正性器出血　107
不整脈　104
不妊症　106
腐敗臭　30
不眠症　105
ふらつく　61
震える　71
風呂　75,92
プロフィール　2
ふわっとする　61
分泌　87
分泌物　55

へ

ヘアピン　46
ペースメーカー　45
ヘモグロビン値　37
減る　69
便　30
　――の色　30
　――の形・硬さ　30
　――の臭い　30
変化なし　13
便通　69
扁桃肥大　107
便秘　9,45,85

ほ

膀胱　38
膀胱炎　**51**,106
放散　12
放射線科　101
放射線技師　102
牧師,病院付きの　103
保険　95,**98**
保健所　81
保険証　98
母語　5

母子手帳　81,92
保証金　95
発作,喘息　89
発作的な　23
発疹　79,91
ボランティア　103
本籍地　7

ま

毎時間　73
毎日　73
前を向く　44
麻疹　108
麻酔　32,59
麻酔医　59
麻酔科　101
まだら　91
待ち合室　55
真っ直ぐ　61
窓口　95,97
まれに　17
慢性の　17
マンモグラフィ　55

み

右向き　31,52
水薬　72
水のような　30
水虫[足白癬]　106
みぞおち　27
緑色　23
緑がかった　30
耳　39
耳がふさがった感じ　64
耳鳴り　64,99
脈　18

む

むくみ　85
向こうずね　43
むち打ち症　106
無痛　17
無痛分娩　81
胸　15

め

明細書　95
目が覚める　69
眼鏡　46
メニエール病　**64**
目のかゆみ　78
目のゴロゴロ　78
めまい　9, 37, **61**, 64
面会時間　65

も

もう一度　3, 11
申し訳ありません　98
持ちもの　65
もちろん　55
ものすごく激しい　23
問題　12, 15

や

薬剤師　102
薬剤投与　**72**
薬剤部長　103
薬疹　106
焼け付くような痛み　51
薬局　97
　——, 院外調剤　72
　——, 病院内の　72
軟らかい　30
和らげる　75

ゆ

誘因　13
郵送　95
ゆっくり　3, 11
指でさす　31
ゆるい　30

よ

用紙　3
腰椎　44
要望　95
用務員　102
予期しない　73
横に手を置く　44
横を向く　44
予定　59
予防接種　**92**
読み書き　5
予約　27
よろける　61

ら

楽にする　19, 24

乱視　107

り

リウマチ・膠原病内科　100
理学療法士　102
リハビリテーション科　101
流行性耳下腺炎　108
領収書　95
両膝　31
療法士　102
緑内障　107
旅行保険　95
臨床工学技士　102
臨床検査技師　102
リンパ腺　91

れ

レントゲン　41, 44

ろ

老年内科　100

わ

わき腹　49

医療英会話
キーワード辞典
そのまま使える16000例文

森島祐子・仁木久恵・Flaminia Miyamasu

**キーワードからピンポイントで答えが見つかる！
和英辞典型の新感覚英会話サポーター**

さまざまな医療場面で必要になる英語表現がキーワードからピンポイントで探せる、これまでになかった和英辞典スタイルの英会話サポートツール。病歴聴取や患者指導、検査、会計などよくある場面・状況については、生きた文例を流れに沿って収載。また「説明する」「大丈夫」「自己負担」など日常よく使う日本語もパッと英語に！

●B6　頁776　2019年　定価：4,180円（本体3,800円＋税10％）［ISBN978-4-260-02813-4］

そのまま使える
病院英語表現
5000
第2版

森島祐子・仁木久恵・Nancy Sharts-Hopko

医療英会話のベストセラー、待望の改訂第2版！

医療英会話を学ぶ読者の圧倒的な支持を得る本書の真骨頂は「シンプル」「丁寧」。第2版でも変わらず、できる限り患者さんに"Yes"か"No"で答えてもらえる表現を紹介し、すべての医療職者を、一方的に話しかけられる恐怖から解放する。今回新たに「リハビリテーション」「医療福祉相談」を追加。病院での英会話に挑戦したい人、今まさに直面している人、さらに磨きをかけたい人、それぞれの新たなスタンダードとなる1冊！

●B6変型　頁472　2013年　定価：3,080円（本体2,800円＋税10％）［ISBN978-4-260-01830-2］

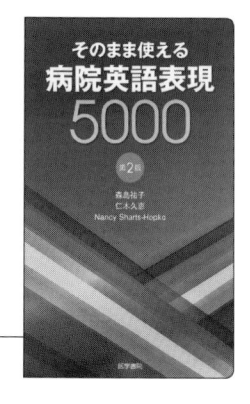

医学書院